IMPROVISATION TECHNIQUE FOR THE LANGUAGE
DEVELOPMENT OF HEARING IMPAIRED CHILDREN

JAYANT VINAYAK PATHAK

TABLE OF CONTENTS

Title	Page No.
Table of Contents	02
List of Abbreviations	03
CHAPTERS	
Chapter 1 Introduction	19
Chapter 2 Review of related literature	37
Chapter 3 Methodology	87
Chapter 4 Analysis and Interpretation	103
Chapter 5 Discussion and Conclusions	169
Chapter 6 Summary	184

LIST OF ABBREVIATIONS

1) Hearing Impaired - H.I.

2) decibel Hearing Loss – dB HL

3) An altered state of consciousness -A.S.C

4) Frequency modulation –FM

5) Cochlear Implant – CI

6) Sensorineural hearing loss –SNHL

7) Audio-verbal therapy –AVT

8) South African Sign Language- SASL

9) American Sign Language -ASL

10) British Sign Language -BSL

11) Deaf or Hard of Hearing - D/HH

12) Pedagogical content knowledge –PCK

13) Individuals with Disabilities Education Act –IDEA

14) Common Core State Standards –CCSS

15) Analysis of Variance –ANOVA

INDEX

CHAPTER 1: Introduction

1.00) Paradigm 22

1.01) Introduction 22

1.02) Personal experience 23

1.03) Need of the study 26

1.04) Nature of the problem 26

1.05) Statement of the problem 26

1.06) Aim and Objectives of the Study 27

    1.06.1 Aim 27

    1.06.2 Objectives 27

1.07) Research questions 27

1.08) Hypothesis 28

1.09) Variables 28

    1.09.1 Independent variable 28

    1.09.2 Dependent variable 28

    1.09.3 Extrinsic variable 28

1.10) Conceptual Definitions 28

    1.10.1 Improvisation technique 29

    1.10.2 Language development 29

    1.10.3 Hearing impaired 29

1.10.4 Hearing loss   29

    1.10.5 Hearing Impaired children   30

    1.10.6 Special school   30

    1.10.7 Special need children   30

1.11) Operational Definitions   30

    1.11.1 Improvisation technique   30

    1.11.2 Language development   30

    1.11.3 Hearing impaired   31

    1.11.4 Hearing loss   31

    1.11.5 Hearing Impaired children: 31

    1.11.6 Special school   31

    1.11.7 Special need children   31

1.12) Assumptions   31

1.13) Significance of the study   31

1.14) Scope, Limitations and Delimitations of the Study   32

    1.14.1 Scope   of the Survey

    1.14.2 Limitations of the Survey

    1.14.3 Delimitations of the Survey

    1.14.4 Scope   of the Experiment

1.14.5 Limitations of the Experiment

1.14.6 Delimitations of the Experiment

1.15) Research Design   34

REFERENCES   35

1.00) Paradigm

Language development of the Hearing Impaired

Personal Experience

Need of the study

Statement of the problem

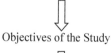

Objectives of the Study

Significance of the study

Research Design

1.01) Introduction:

Hearing is one of the important factors which decide the 'quality' of our life. Taxing impairment has adverse effects on leading a 'quality' life in the affected individuals. If not attended in time, it comes in the way of the individual utilizing one's own potentials to the maximum. It may be in terms of speech and language development, educational achievement, vocational placement. [1]

The occurrence of other disabilities in combination with diminished hearing creates additional learning problems, which significantly add to the complexity of educating the student who is

22

deaf. The three additional disabilities most often reported in children who are deaf are learning disabilities, intellectual disabilities, and emotional/behavioral disabilities.[2]

1.02) Personal Experience

The researcher observed the difference in Hearing Impaired students' communication among themselves and with normal people.   The hearing impaired students are diffident in communication with normal people, but feel free and comfortable with the Hearing Impaired students. The researcher himself tried various forms of dramatics for providing H.I. Students the opportunity of expression that would give them confidence. He got the opportunity of trying the drama as project work for Diploma in Special Education University of Pune. It was written for normal children. However the play was to be presented by hearing impaired girls from Integration Units. They through their gestures and body language established communication with the audience effectively, as if they presented the dialogues in normal Marathi. This experience brought to the notice a very special endeavor of hearing impaired students. It was a very notable experience of sharing drama practices and improvisation with these H.I. students having a moderate loss.

Researcher had completed his Diploma in special education.

Project: Participation in drama competition with H.I. girl students, studying in 5th to10th STD.

Methodology: Use of a written script with improvisation technique.

1) To introduce the technique of a drama.

2) To learn the communication with co-actor and audience simultaneously.

3) To practice the formal conversation with other person.

Objectives: 1) to test the improvisation technique for improvement in spoken language.

2) To check the verbal mastery with the help of the dialogues.

3) To introduce the dramatics among the H.I.schoolgirl students.

Sampling: the group of high school students having hearing loss 80dB to 110dB, age between 11yrs to 16yrs. They were from different economical and social strata. Every student has her own style of learning, level of language development, style of pronunciation, comprehension and expression. All students were from integration unit. In this unit the H.I.student has opportunity to interact with normal hearing students; teachers help them in language development with practicing one to one communication, while teaching. Students are free to express themselves through conversation, experiments and doing actions wherever they want.

Selection of a script: the subject in the script was related with the emotional and familiar world of the selected age group. In the preface of the script the author mentions "generally the high school students have high artistic potentials to express themselves in performing arts. That is why this script has less importance in drapery, makeup, settings, lights, music etc."[3] The script demands more on imagination and spontaneous acting style. It is a part of experimental theatre; it gives opportunity to creativity in H.I.student through live and verbal presentation.

As a director, the researcher broadly divided the script in two parts: (1) the speech part and (2) dramatization/presentation the improvisation technique part.

For the first part every student was corrected in speech using her individual hearing aid, the dialogues were practiced with correct pauses, pitch variation, intensity with emotions accordingly.

For the second part the improvisation technique was practiced for every scene in the script.

Improvisation is a stimulating teaching strategy which promotes cooperation, collaboration, self- control, goal-oriented learning also as emotional intelligence skills. Improvisation bridges the gap between printed-book dialogues and natural usage, and can also help to bridge an identical gap between the classroom and real world situations by providing insights into the way to handle difficult situations. Drama and songs, for instance, strengthen the bond between thought and expression in language, and offer good listening practice. If Improvisation is taken into account as pedagogies within the sense of being a part of the eclectic approach to teaching, then it can become a main aid within the acquisition of communicative competence.

Improvisation activities facilitate the sort of language behavior that ought to cause fluency, and if it's accepted that the learners want to find out language so as to form themselves understood within the language, then, improvisation does indeed, further this end. One of the best advantages to be gained from the utilization of drama, songs and games is that students become more confident in their use of language by experiencing the language in operation. Improvisation encourages adaptability, fluency, and communicative competence. It puts language into context, and by giving learners experience of success in real-life situations it should arm them confidently for tackling the planet outside the classroom[4]. Improvisation encourages students to mobilize their vocabulary, answer grammatical and syntactical accuracy, and develop cultural and social awareness, and gain confidence and fluency. Through constant repetition of words and phrases, they become conversant in them and are ready to say them with increasing fluency by encouraging self- expression; drama, especially, motivates students to use language confidently and creatively[5]. Improvisation enables the students to flex their emotional, mental also as physical muscles during a safe and controlled setting. the students will develop an increasing facility to satisfy changing and unknown stimuli with immediate responses. Improvisation activities give the scholar several avenues to self-awareness[6].

Observations: The students enjoyed the drama practices and the performance. They showed a good example of a team work and collaborating activity. Everyone tried to learn new words verbally and expressively. Everyone tried to know her character in the play; it was a good co-operative exercise with each other. Each student was confident about her role and was eager to enact .The basic technique of drama was introduced to the team including how to stand before the audience, use of breathing during speech, the movements on the stage, use of acting area, correct facial expressions, eye contacts with the co-actors, composition sense, entries and exists, tendencies towards the actors and audience, use of properties and musical instruments.

After the performance everyone was eager to talk and share her experience with each other and their parents. Parents were pleased and satisfied with the process of practice and performance. The process of improvisation helps the students to raise their confidence level. They tried to communicate more people. They like to interact with unknown person also. Their informal communication with others became more free and confident. Some of the students talked their experience with their relatives also. Very long time after their performance, they remembered their dialogues with emotions, their actions, the movements they performed in their presentation.

The team got 3rd prize in that competition.

Summary: The process of improvisation and drama shows us a number of things about the ways in which the children learn the language. It is natural to them for jump from one thought to another, and to make the different types of connections that are seldom in textbooks and within formal teaching-learning process in classrooms. The younger children were more curious and fear-free to do the experiments with language.

1.03) Need of the study

The researcher is working in a secondary school in Pune. The researcher got the opportunity through the interactions to observe the emotional and cognitive world of the students. The researcher also works as a teacher educator in B.Ed. College of special education and has to guide teacher trainees for their classroom lessons. The observation of the lessons made the researcher very uneasy due to the struggle of Hearing Impaired students at times, fruitless for expressing themselves in language known to normal students and adults. Also the effort for a very long time taken by the parents and the teachers of these students motivates the researcher to undertake the study.

1.04) Nature of the problem:

Normally there are number of techniques for language development. The sequence to acquire the language is listening, speech, reading, and writing. But the Hearing Impaired children have barrier at the first stage. Hence the obstacles in their language learning were investigated through the questionnaires by teachers and parents. The effectiveness of improvisation technique for language development can be checked by experimentation.

For testing the effectiveness, experimentation was must. To investigate difficulties in language development a survey was necessary. Recognizing these needs into consideration the problem was specified.

1.05) Statement of the problem:

In the light of the personal experience strengthened through reading the researcher stated the problem as under:-

Conducting a survey of the present methods of language teaching applied by teachers from special schools and parents of hearing impaired students with a view to overcoming the difficulties in language development and applying the improvisation technique for language development of hearing impaired students from residential schools and testing its effectiveness

from Pune city and a suburb of Pune.

1.06) Aim and Objectives of the study:

1.06.1) Aim:-

To explore the language development of hearing impaired student with a moderate and severe hearing loss.

1.06.2) Objectives:-

(1) To investigate difficulties in language development faced by the hearing impaired students, their teachers and parents.

(2)To examine the present ways and methods of language teaching applied by teachers from special school and parents of hearing impaired students with a view to overcoming the difficulties in language development.

(3) To develop The Improvisation programme for hearing impaired students.

(4) To test the effectiveness of improvisation technique in language development of hearing impaired students.

1.07) Survey Related Major research questions:

1) What are the difficulties in language development of hearing impaired child?

2) Why do these difficulties occur?

3) What are the present ways and methods applied by teachers and parents to overcome these difficulties?

4) Which processes are important for language development of hearing impaired?

1.08) Hypotheses:

Experiment Related:

(1) There will be significant difference in pre test and post test scores for language development in the experimental group.

(2)There will be no significant difference in pre test and post test scores for language development in the control group..

(3)There will be a positive gain in the language development of experimental group as compared to that in control group.

1.09) Variables

The following variables are found in the present research study.

1.09.1) Independent Variable : In this research study, 'Improvisation Technique' is considered as an independent variable as this technique is supposed to be responsible for bringing about change

1.09.2) Dependent Variables :In this research study, 'language development of students having moderate loss and moderately severe hearing loss' is considered as dependent variable as it is the outcome of the change brought about by introduction of an independent variable.

1.09.3) Extrinsic Variables : In this research study, 'School environment, teaching methods of the teachers, interaction of students with other students and their parents, interaction of parents with school 'are considered as extrinsic variables as the above mentioned factors may affect changes in on the dependent variables. These factors are not measured in the study, may increase or decrease the magnitude of the relationship between independent and dependent variables.

1.10) Conceptual definitions:

1.10.1 Improvisation technique[7]: Improvisation is the practice of acting, reacting, verbal expressions in real time and in response to one's immediate environment and emotions. This may result in new thought process, new signs and symbols, rather new way to act. This occurs effectively when the student has a profound intuitive and technical knowledge of the necessary skills.

1.10.2 Language development[8]: Language development is the process by which children come to understand and communicate language during early childhood.

1.10.3 Hearing impaired[9]: Hearing loss is typically categorized as normal, slight, mild, moderate, moderately severe, severe, profound or total, depending on the hearing impaired person's ability to hear sounds clearly. A person with normal hearing should be able to hear sounds measured at 0 to 15 decibels and higher. Those with slight hearing loss should be able to hear sounds measured at 16 to 25 decibels and higher. Those with mild hearing loss should be able to hear sounds measured at 26 to 40 decibels and higher. Those with moderate hearing loss should be able to hear sounds measured at 41 to 55 decibels and higher. Those with moderately severe hearing loss should be able to hear sounds measured at 56 to 70 decibels and higher .Those with severe impairment may only be able to hear sounds measured at 71 to 90 decibels and higher. Persons so hearing impaired that they can't hear sounds at all are considered profound deaf.

1.10.4 Hearing loss[10]:

Degree of hearing loss	Hearing loss range (dB HL)
Normal	0 to 15
Slight	16 to 25
Mild	26 to 40
Moderate	41 to 55

Moderately severe	56 to 70
Severe	71 to 90
Profound	91+

1.10.5 Hearing Impaired children[11]:

students in school having a range of mild to moderate hearing loss and moderately severe hearing loss.

1.10.6 Special school[12]:

A special school is a school accommodating students who have special educational needs due to learning difficulties, physical disabilities or behavioral problems.

1.10.7 Special need children[13]:

the children who require assistance for disabilities that may be physical, medical, mental, or psychological.

1.11) Operational definitions:

1.11.1 Improvisation technique:

Improvisation is the practice of acting, singing, talking and reacting, of making and creating, in the moment and in response to the stimulus of one's immediate environment and inner feelings. This can result in the invention of new thought patterns, new practices, new structures or symbols, and/or new ways to act. This invention cycle occurs most effectively when the practitioner has a thorough intuitive and technical understanding of the necessary skills and concerns within the improvised domain.

1.11.2 Language development:

Language development is the process by which children comprehend the language and is measured by Educational progress test i.e. baseline test made by Government of Maharashtra (Maharashtra Pradhikaran Parishad, 2017)

1.11.3 Hearing impaired: The children having moderate to moderately severe hearing loss.

1.11.4 Hearing loss: The hearing loss of 71dB and above.

1.11.5 Hearing Impaired children: students learning in special and residential schools having moderate hearing loss and moderately severe hearing loss.

1.11.6 Special school: a school accommodating students who have special educational needs due to their moderately severe hearing loss.

1.11.7 Special need children: Children having severe hearing loss studying in residential special primary school.

1.12) Assumptions:

(1) Language of hearing impaired is acquired[14].

(2) Training improves the performance[15].

1.13) Significance of the study:

Improvisation has high potential of inbuilt spontaneity with respect to content, theme, communication skills. The factors such as self motivation, confidence, listening capacity, and observation of the participant help a lot for presentation of improvisation. A lack of hearing adversely affects language learning, creating a major obstacle in expressing one's thoughts, feelings, and emotions[16]. Taking into consideration the experience of the project work cited above and the experience of using the technique of improvisation it was felt intensely that language development of hearing impaired students with a moderate and moderately severe hearing loss can be achieved through Improvisation.

The use of Improvisation in the organization of learning experiences would reduce the hurdles in understanding the concepts. It will also help in the process of language development is a guess and if is found correct would bring in transformation in the teaching learning of hearing impaired students. This indicates the direction of the effective and efficient modifications in instructional system of hearing impaired students. In the end the language development would be facilitated and in turn would facilitate their entire learning.

1.14) Scope, limitations and delimitations of the study

1.14.1) Scope of the Survey covers the following:

The survey was undertaken for the parents and teachers of hearing impaired students from the special deaf schools of Pune area.

1.14.2) Limitations of the Survey:

Only hearing impaired students from special and residential schools were selected for the experiment.

1.14.3) Delimitation of the Survey:

For the survey, the hearing impaired students from the normal schools, integration units, and non-residential schools were not selected for the study.

1.14.4) Scope of the Experimental study covers the following:

The experimental study was conducted in the special residential schools with the students having moderate and severe hearing loss. The hearing impaired students of standard first, second and third were selected for the experiment. Two schools out of four from suburbs were selected.

1.14.5) Limitations of the Experimental study:

Conclusions made from the programme were based the experiment conducted in the academic year 2016-17.

1.14.6) Delimitation of the Experimental study:

Researcher decided to implement Pretest Post test experimental design to examine the eeffectiveness of improvisation technique in language development. Sample which was selected for the experimental and control group was from residential deaf schools from a suburb of Pune. These schools were selected by researcher as the required sample was from equal socio, economical and educational background.

1.15) Method of the Study

The objectives of the present research are as follows-

(1) To investigate difficulties in language development faced by the hearing impaired students, their teachers and parents.

(2)To examine the present ways and methods of language teaching applied by teachers from special school and parents of hearing impaired students with a view to overcoming the difficulties in language development.

In Objectives One and two, researcher wanted to understand status of difficulties in language development and applied teaching methods to overcome these difficulties by parents and teachers from the special deaf schools of Pune area. Therefore, researcher chose Survey method. Survey methods describe, compare, contrast, classify, analyze and interpret the events that constitute various fields of inquiry. Surveys gather data at a particular point in time with the intention of describing the nature of existing conditions, or identifying standards against which existing conditions can be compared, or determining the relationships that exist between specific events.

(3) To develop The Improvisation programme for hearing impaired students.

To achieve Objective three, researcher designed 'Training Program'. Planning and implementation report as elaborated in Chapter 3.

(4) To test the effectiveness of improvisation technique in language development of hearing impaired students.

To achieve Objective four, researcher decided on experimental method of study. The experimental method allows researcher to deliberately control and manipulate the control and manipulate the conditions which determines the outcome in which the researcher is interested in. An experiment involves making a change in the value of one variable – called the independent

variable i.e. the input variable and observing the effect of that change on another variable –
called the dependent variable i.e. the outcome variable.

Research Design:

The researcher is going to test the effectiveness of the technique of Improvisation in language
development of hearing impaired student. So the pretest posttest of the experimental and control
group design is to be selected.

Taking into consideration the spread of population of students with moderate hearing loss and
moderately severe loss, the random selection of the sample for control and experiment will be
difficult. So equivalent groups of students will be selected and distributed for control and
experimental treatment.[17]

CHAPTER 1:REFERNCES

1) https://www.ncbi.nlm.nih.gov/pmc/articles/PMC3393360/

2) https://www.ericdigests.org/1998-2/deaf.htm

ERIC Identifier: ED414666,Publication Date: 1997-08-00,Author: Pollack, B. J.,
Source: ERIC Clearinghouse on Disabilities and Gifted Education Reston VA.

3) Vijay Tendulkar, Patalachya Poriche Lagin, Mauj Prakashan Grih, Girgaon, Mumbai 1987

4) https://files.eric.ed.gov/fulltext/EJ420165.pdf

Paul Davies, The Use of Drama in English Language Teaching

5) http://publish.ucc.ie/journals/scenario/2013/02, VolumeVII, ISSN 1649-8526

6) http://202.15.16.209/Articles/Boudreault-Drama.html

Chris Boudreault ,The Benefits of Using Drama in the ESL/EFL Classroom

7) Editors: Frederic, Agnes F. Vandome, John McBrewster,Improvisation ,VDM Publishing,
2009,ISBN 6130094795, 9786130094799

8) Wikipedia

9) Wikipedia

10) American Speech Language Hearing Association

11) World Health Organisation

12) Cambridge dictionary

13) Collins dictionary

14) core.ac.uk

15) researchgate.net

16) https://www.ncbi.nlm.nih.gov/books/NBK207837/?report

Dobie RA, Van Hemel S, editors. Hearing Loss: Determining Eligibility for Social Security Benefits. National Research Council (US) Committee on Disability Determination for Individuals with Hearing Impairments; Washington (DC): National Academies Press (US); 2004.

17) Best W. John and Kahn V. James- Research in Education (10th Edition), PHI Learning Private Limited, 2009. ISBN 978-81-203-3563-9

INDEX

CHAPTER 2: Review of Related Literature

2.00) Paradigm   38

2.01) Introduction   38

2.02) Surveys   39

2.03) Observations   83

2.04) Characteristics of the present study   84

REFERENCES   86

2.00) Paradigm

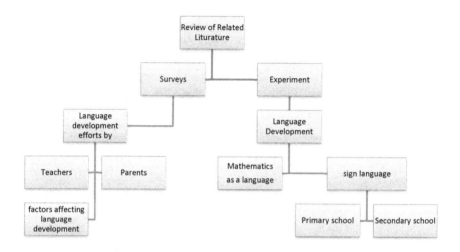

2.01) Introduction:

With the decision of studying the use of Improvisation in the language learning of H.I .students it was but natural to search the previous work in the related area.

In Indian Educational Research Abstracts published by NCERT, the theories of language learning and the methods of teaching languages to H.I.student were the three basic dimensions that were pursued. It was found that the language learning of H.I. students and the use of improvisation as a technique in language development were not mentioned .Then the internet was approached.

The researcher noted down the efforts made by the researchers in the area of language development of hearing impaired students .The common focus of these researches was the speech of the hearing impaired child. The language development of a child is observable by speech. But is it a single way or the only indication to study the language gaining? It is seen from the researches in foreign countries that stress is on empowering the natural instrument i.e. the ear; through cochlear implantation .The cost of the surgery is not within the reach of common man. Inclusive education for equity is our national commitment. This necessitates the search of methods for H.I .students leading to language learning with a minimal cost. One such direction for developing a new approach to H.I. student's language learning was found in the use of dramatics. Skills such as listening, clarity of thought, confidence and performing instantly and spontaneously is considered to help develop the language. These skills are developed through dramatics as was revealed through these research studies[1]. So through these studies the researcher got the empirical base for his own conjecture. Improvisation being the subset of dramatics would accelerate language learning of the H.I. students.

The researcher viewed improvisation as an altered state of consciousness (A.S.C.) in which students routinely and voluntarily enters. There are 14 dimensions of subjective experiences which characterize Altered State of Consciousness namely-attention, perception, imagery and fantasy, inner speech, memory, higher level thought process, meaning or significance of experience, emotional feeling and expression, level of arousal, self control, suggestibility, body image and sense of personal identity[2].

In short the review provided the logical and empirical base for the researcher's conjecture.

2.02) Surveys:

The deaf population in India is the largest in the world which is more than 18 million. According to the latest data, the number of deaf schools in India is more than 550[3]. In the yester years, deaf children were a curse for their parents, relatives and even teachers. But, many changes have happened in the society. At present, the importance of deaf education is increasing. The awareness is spreading in different parts of the country. However, the deaf population in India is neglecting the importance of education because of various reasons. Therefore, greater awareness regarding this matter is essential among the Indian deaf population. Problems generally faced by most of the deaf students at their special schools are: Sign language is the most prominent communication medium for deaf people. But, the usage of sign language is very insignificant in many schools in India. The schools force the students to sit in the class and ask them to listen to gestures and lip reading of their teachers. The biggest problem faced by the deaf children and their teachers is the non availability of a uniform sign language. The language development is extremely difficult due to the lack of a uniform sign language[4].

Parents of Deaf must Learn Sign Language.

Parents must communicate with the deaf kids effectively, which is expected for providing general awareness to the deaf kid. Sign language helps parents to communicate with their deaf kid very easily.

Most deaf children start their education in normal schools. So, they will not get training in sign language. Lip reading is the only option before them and they try to understand things by observing lip reading. But, lip reading is not so effective for understanding things clearly. As a result, most deaf students are not able to write alphabet without mistakes. In such a way, they complete their plus two and join degree courses. They face lots of difficulties due to improper training in schools. A small percentage of deaf children in India use early intervention centers. However, these types of centers do not teach sign language during the primary years of the students. As a result, the deaf children fail to understand the concept of abstract nouns.

Difficulties to read:

Reading is not enjoyable for most deaf children. They face difficulties to understand imagery, idioms, phrases, etc. Therefore, reading is enjoyable for only a small percentage of deaf individuals[5]. They are also not able to express their ideas in written language. The number of deaf children who can write sentences without mistakes is also very less. Most of them cannot enjoy poems because they contain idioms, imagery, etc.

Most of them are not able to remember what they studied in the class rooms because they are not able to relate things and situations with other situations. They have only very a smaller amount vocabulary. The vocabulary improvement is also not done properly in school days. Usually, they learn by heart and reproduce it on the papers during exams.

(4)A case study

Findings: A newborn is identified as having sensorineural deafness. The parents are normal in hearing and unaware of sign language. A hearing aid is not medically indicated. They have a few months to decide whether to opt for a CI.

(5) The article

Method: early diagnosis and early intervention of crucial importance.

Findings: the importance of allowing deaf children to acquire sign language from an early age. It reveals that the critical/sensitive period hypothesis for language acquisition can be applied to specific language aspects of spoken language as well as sign languages (i.e. phonology, grammatical processing and syntax). (6) The rationale for choosing sign language as communication medium and language of instruction for deaf learners.

(7) Introduction

In areas with a large Deaf community, almost everyone knows or has met someone who is Deaf or Hard of Hearing (D/HH) but very few people understand the obstacles that deaf or hard of hearing persons face.

(8)The case study is one of six short case studies which explore the activity that has taken place in the first year of Time to Shine, Scotland's Youth Arts Strategy.

(9) Sample Size: A total of 20 young people participated in the empirical research, including 7 young people who participated in in-depth qualitative interviews.

(10) Abstract: the article is based on a qualitative case study of teachers' conceptions of improvisation in teaching. Empirical data are master student teachers' texts (transcripts, reflections) based on observations and interviews of practicing teachers.

Observations

From the report of https://worldwidescience.org/topicpages/h/hearing+deaf+children.html refers that:

(1)Group study:

A study of 213 mothers and 213 fathers of of hearing impaired children was executed.

Method used to observe was an array of different questionnaires.

.

41

Findings: The child's communicative capability makes for a more sound prediction than its language.

Findings: The results show that high parental stress is associated with repeated socioemotional problems in the children, thus emphasize the importance of early intervention. Child development seems to profits enormously from a resource-oriented support model. Results also shows that: parents with additional disabled children are principally stressed.[6]

(2)Method: A controlled longitudinal study.

Findings:

A controlled longitudinal study shows that the mother's sensitivity to her deaf or hard of hearing child is responsible for the child's linguistic development between ages 2 and 3.

The mother's sensitivity to the child's signs and an appropriate placing of impulses for interaction and development were mainly projecting of the deaf children's linguistic development. The sensitivity, appropriate change and interaction order seem to assume special importance for the condition of "deafness."

Early diagnosis and intervention seem to be the best precautionary plan against stress for the parents of hearing impaired children.

The child's socioemotional development is improved in parent–child constellations in which parents adjust their communication behavior to their deaf child's form of communication than with parents who do not.

The child's hearing status, child age, and the language used to communicate with the child seem to be comparatively poor indicators for child development. Particularly with regard to the language used with the child, it is to state that "the method of communication on its own is not an indicator in the development of language, cognition and social skills".

Findings:

The deaf parents with deaf children show interactive qualities in their interactive behavior as compare to those of hearing parents with hearing children. That is why deaf children of deaf parents experience better socioemotional and age-appropriate cognitive development. Also do not run a high risk of behavioral problems because of their hearing loss. The difference between deaf children of deaf parents and deaf children of hearing parents becomes more and more indistinct as soon as the schools offer sign language in addition to oral methods.

Discussion: One of the particularly significant findings is that the child's communicative competence has an effect on both parental stress experience and the child's development, whereas the modality of that competence has no effect. We thus find less parenting and relationship stress in families with a communicatively competent child, with the child's development progressing better than in families without this condition. This finding may be important even though we have no differentiated information about the exact use of signing with the children, meaning that the distinction between spoken language and signing in this study may be too restricted. But in following up on this finding, which has been reproduced many times by now, educational practice has the important task of exploring the communicative potential and circumstances of each individual deaf or hard of hearing child and his/her family and of adapting its support on the basis of that knowledge so as to achieve the best possible communicative competence in the child regardless of modality[7].

Deaf children who are not provided with a sign language early in their development are at risk of linguistic deprivation; they may never be confident in any language. These children are socially and emotionally isolated. Deafness makes a child helpless to abuse these children are socially and emotionally isolated. Deafness makes a child helpless to abuse, and linguistic deprivation compounds the abuse because the child is less able to report it. Parents rely on professionals as guides in making responsible choices in raising and educating their deaf children.

Findings:

The pressure of ignore is likely to be higher for deaf children, who have reduced access to language, are often cut off socially, and are already at risk for worse psychological and cognitive development that can affect academic inequality also.

Findings:

There is indication of greater depression severity in deaf adult patients. Those felt left out from family communication during childhood compared to deaf adult patients who had better communication with their parents.

Findings:

Isolating a child and denying emotional sensitivity to a child go hand-in-hand with not maintaining an environment for the child to build a solid foundation in a language. All children need regular and frequent exposure to an accessible language during the critical period between birth and 3 or 4 years old or they risk linguistic deprivation. Linguistic deficiency inhibits ease in any language and correlates with a range of poor cognitive and academic outcomes. Many deaf children who are raised using only spoken language do not receive enough access to aural information to develop language. These children have cognitive deficits associated with those faculties that require a firm base in a first language.

The child without social communication does not have the chance to develop the social and cognitive skills, which are fundamentals for education and for assuming a creative and satisfying position in society.

Findings:

In deaf children with no language delays, the structural design of the brain is protected and social communication is strong. These children have been found not to have an issue with sustained attention, which is an important cognitive skill for being able to function in an educational setting, and this is one reason why signing deaf children do better academically than nonsigning ones.

If a child is exposed regularly and repeatedly to a language and picks up that language naturally without precise training and exercise, the language qualifies as accessible to that child. On the other hand, if a child is exposed regularly and frequently to a language but does not pick it up even after precise training and exercise, the language is possibly inaccessible to that child. As hearing loss can affect access to spoken language, which is a biological limitation on language exposure, so decisions to exclude exposure to sign language can affect access to language, which can lead to social limitation.

Findings:

It is important that sign languages are accessible to all deaf children, providing a sign language as early as possible is the more reliable way to ensure a deaf child's language development and prevent linguistic deprivation .The harm of failing to reassure language development is compounded by the fact that this particular neglect increases deaf children's risk for other maltreatments and decreases their ability to report these maltreatments.

Language development, a critical part of overall cognitive development, is under most circumstances a naturally acquired object of human interaction. Hence, when human language interaction is absent, the result is severe cognitive deficits.

One misunderstanding is that language is taken as counterpart to speech. This assumption is out-of-date and comes with severe consequences. Language is a cognitive faculty that can be manifested in more than one modality: oral–aural, realized as speech, and manual–visual, realized as sign. The two modalities are equal cognitive citizens, so to speak; language development is modality-independent and people can express themselves fully in either modality. Evidence supporting this comes from research in many areas, including linguistic analysis, first language acquisition, neurology in matters of language pathologies, and language processing, as well as expressive capacity.

Deaf children who acquire a sign language from birth do not risk language delay or deficit, their reading abilities are better than deaf children from other backgrounds. There is a strong correlation between better signing skills and better print literacy in number of studies. With continued means of direct communication apt to the individual (sign, speech, or writing) and with apt accommodations such as amplifications, frequency modulation (FM) systems, captioning, or interpreting services throughout schooling, deaf children can grow up to be creative adults.

Responsibility for Language Deprivation and Neglect

There is greatly increasing social consciousness of sign languages and the benefits of visual access to language for deaf children. Increasing training and awareness of language acquisition in two modes, aural and visual, also needs to be a main concern in the social services and in medical professions.

Findings: Conclusion

All deaf children should be enabled to acquire a sign language through early, frequent, and regular exposure; failure to do so greatly increases the risk of cognitive harm and thus constitutes neglect. Because acquiring sign language does no harm and carries no risk, it is much safer for deaf children to have early exposure to it than the alternative of an oral approach, which carries a strong risk of inadequate exposure to language.

The right to language is well-known principle in society, which is becoming more applicable to deaf children and their right to whole and natural language. Sign language ensures this right because of its accessible nature. Deaf children have a legal right to language, and they have a right to grow up bilingually, using a sign language and a spoken language (often in the written form of that language)[8].

3) Abstract from the survey
https://www.researchgate.net/publication/278732836_Should_All_Deaf_Children_Learn_Sign_Language refers the following

Findings:Every year, 10 000 infants are born in the United States with sensorineural deafness. The incidence of sensorineural deafness is similar in most high-income countries and is higher in some low-income countries. Many infants become deaf in early age i.e. before 2 years.

Every year, 10 000 infants are born in the United States with sensorineural deafness. The incidence of sensorineural deafness is similar in most high-income strata and is higher in some low-income strata. Many more infants become deaf in early age i.e. before 2 years. Experts differ that a child must be exposed to an reachable language on a regular and frequent basis before 5 years of age to develop full language ability.

The approach to hearing restoration are being applied to younger children at increasing rates; some estimates indicate that more than one-half of US children with early-onset deafness have received a Cochlear Implant.

Findings: Children with CIs require intensive rehabilitation throughout childhood to learn to communicate orally. With this training, some children become better oral communicators than others. Some experts suggest that all deaf children, with or without a CI, should be taught a sign language[9].

(4)A CASE STUDY: A newborn is identified as having sensorineural deafness. The parents have normal hearing and not aware of sign language. A hearing aid is not medically indicated. They have a less time to decide whether to decide on for a CI.

Parents are often judgmental about a child's deafness through their own hearing status. Hearing parents normally believe of hearing impairment as a disability. Their views are shaped by their need to share their own language and culture with their child.

A deaf child born to hearing parents and incapable to gain significant speech recognition from hearing aids will typically meet the criteria for early cochlear implantation. The US Food and Drug Administration approved the multichannel CI for children in 1990. Almost 100 000 children have used CIs successfully to expand spoken language. However, a CI can enable strong spoken language only when used with thorough auditory-oral coverage in extended, salient, and child-initiated interactions. Without a full linguistic and auditory experience, the effects of deafness-associated deficiency can ruin the spoken language learning process before it begins.

The timing of intervention is very critical. An infant's nervous system is genetically predisposed to accept only a limited range of potential stimuli to drive the developmental learning of language. Experiences that produce language occur in a "biologically expensive" period in which neural circuits are undecided yet amenable to commitment. During this sensitive period, use of neural circuits generates the impulse traffic that differentiates neural development. If a child misses the needed experiences within an optimal time frame, essential elements in that child's emergent language, either spoken or signed, may be missing.

Early experience with sign language may support a child's participation in the foundation of language learning, for example, by enabling joint attention. However, an important limitation should be considered. The use of any residual hearing should be maximized. Data from a probable, national trial in progress signify that verbal language learned before cochlear implantation is associated with accelerated rates of spoken language learning after implantation.

For a child who receives a CI, the timely activation of the device begins a fuller experience with sound. Dependence on sign language over an extended period of time may adversely affect the child's capacity to learn spoken language after cochlear implantation. Expanded, insufficient auditory input that fails to support spoken language learning at age-appropriate rates is related to gaps in speech and language after cochlear implantation. Importantly, even extensive rehabilitative efforts will not produce the language complexity that can be achieved by exposure to spoken language during sensitive periods of development.

A child's skill to effectively acquire spoken language requires a framework of rich, bidirectional communication with language mentors and interest in an oral language environment. Because the CI is designed to equip a child with skills to communicate in a hearing world, we strongly promote for educational programs that allow children to access the pragmatics of spoken language in interactions with their hearing peers.

https://www.researchgate.net/

Publication/278732836_Should_All_Deaf_Children_Learn_Sign_Language reports in a CASE STUDY:

Sign language is very precious for deaf children, but families need time and space to adjust and come to provisions with everything that is happening to them and to the reality of being the parents of a deaf child.

The hearing parent of a profoundly deaf son with bilateral CIs has had his CIs for 5 years. He has age-appropriate oral/aural language skills and attends a conventional primary school with support from a specialist teacher for the deaf. Even with his CIs and spoken language skills, he remains deaf and always will be. CIs have the same restrictions as other artificial hearing devices; they are helpful in close range with slight background noise. Given these limitations, it is necessary that we have a means of communicating with him, and he with us, when hearing is not an option. Research suggests that speech reading can be a useful additional tool. An alternate form of communication is therefore needed.

Another important factor is that the level of signing support accessible to families depends on the location in which they live. Signing clubs can also be distant places for hearing families.

Deaf children are given access to both oral/aural and signed language to facilitate them to make their own choice when old enough to do so. This stance seems entirely reasonable, maximize the opportunities available. It would seem rational to encourage the family of a deaf child to sign with their child. It is essential that these families are given the support they need to do so, however. This support includes time and space to psychologically alter to the new world in which they find themselves as well as practical and/or financial support.

There are 3 powerful reasons to learn both signed and written/spoken language.

First, a speech only approach risks linguistic deficiency at a vital period of development. The sign language and beginners reading are visually easily available to the deaf child. The bilingual approach guarantees that the child will develop linguistic proficiency.

Second, bilingualism is advantageous. Bilingual children display better mental flexibility and cognitive control as well as more creative thinking. These profits extend to social as well as academic settings.

Third, sign language development correlates positively with written and spoken language development. No evidence has been found that the use of a visual language positively affects the outcome of cochlear implantation. It seems that early and frequently experience to sign language may provide a 'framework' for language development in hearing impaired children.

In most crucial period i.e. from birth to 3 years of age, a deaf child needs to be part of linguistic inputs.

Academic language development is what we suppose of children in school, the language that children must both access and exhibit knowledge in. Being able to communicate in sign language with the teacher and with classmates affords the deaf child the socially and intellectually engaged interaction that comprises so much of the school day.

This social development is decisive to students' ability to learn and to their moral and emotional development. As the deaf child grows, in spite of the family a large amount of the child's time is spent away from home. With sign language, the deaf child is able to go through various social situations and communities without difficulty and not be restricted to communicating only with family and friends, as is often the case for deaf children who have no knowledge of sign language. All deaf children should be taught a sign language as soon as their hearing status is determined[10].

Language learners have a range of problems, particularly with literacy, whereas signing hearing impaired children, with or without a CI, achieve better on literacy and cognitive skills that require language foundation, in spite of whether their parents are hearing or deaf. They experience overall advantage with no drawbacks if they continue to sign while oral training is still in progress. Sign and speech works simultaneously with each other. The fact is, acquiring a firm basis in a sign language gives the child the base upon which to build skills in reading and speaking a second language.

Raising a deaf child with a sign language and spoken language at a time requires learning a sign language. But raising a deaf child only orally requires daily training in vocalization and speech-reading right through childhood.

Various combinations of speech, gestures, and elementary signing can help in family communication, and such systems have some similarities to natural language. However, these systems are no substitute for genuine language, nor do they allow the child to communicate with others outside the family. If families permit their deaf children to interact with signing deaf adults, these deaf adults will serve as the resource that allows first language acquisition to develop naturally. Deaf children also have to interact with other deaf children who sign. One can find these language and social opportunities through community support groups such as deaf support groups, local deaf and hard-of-hearing community centers.

The family can begin sign language classes as soon as the deafness is diagnosed. Some family members may become fluent signers, while others may always feel uncomfortable at signing;

however the fact that the family communicates with the child. Deaf children who sign with their hearing mothers show early language fluency similar to hearing children of the same age despite variability in the mothers' signing abilities.

At first 3 years of age, a deaf child needs to be part of a language and cognitive ecosystem in which clear linguistic input and rich interaction with print prepare the child for both the possession of basic interpersonal communication skills and for academic language development. By acquiring sign language in crucial period, the child can build up theory of mind and achieve the requisite domestication of vision (e.g., eye tracking for reading) to be ready for schooling.

Academic language development is what we anticipate of children in school, the language that children must both access and demonstrate knowledge in. Being able to communicate in sign language with the teacher and with classmates affords the deaf child the socially and intellectually engaged interaction that comprises so much of the school day.

Deaf infants need exposure to good signing models (i.e., people using a sign language with all of its grammatical richness), not just too good speakers. Various combinations of speech, gestures, can help in family communication, because such systems have some structural similarities to natural language. But, these systems are neither substitute for language, nor do they allow communicating with others outside the family. If families permit their deaf children to interact with signing deaf adults, these deaf adults will serve as the resource that allows first language acquisition to develop naturally. Deaf children also need to interact with other deaf children who sign. One can find these language and social opportunities through community support groups such as deaf advocacy groups, local deaf and hard-of-hearing community centers, and local and/or state deaf services bureaus.

Parents are misguided that the best way for their child to acquire spoken language is to raise them without sign language. In many cases, parents are advised that sign is to be chosen only as a last option, and that great effort should be devoted instead to the acquisition of speech.

CI is now the treatment of choice in the medical sciences for most children with sensorineural hearing loss (SNHL), and sign language is seen as both a barrier to learning speech and a symptom of treatment failure. The most frequent recommendation is to isolate deaf children from sign language environments during the important years of first language acquisition. The factors involved in CI success are not well understood, although age of the patient, onset of deafness, family socioeconomical and educational background, are relevant. Many implanted children who are born deaf or become deaf in the first few years of life experience little to no success in language acquisition with a CI. They turn to sign language after the early critical period. Unfortunately, these children are under the risk of never having completely fluent use of either a spoken or a sign language. Not fulfilling the language needs of deaf children can adversely affect to their psycho-social health, putting them at risk for depression, behavioral problems, and social disorders. Long term, language access is critical for the participation of deaf people in preventive health, education, mental health, and social relationships. Additionally, failure to acquire language in the early critical years results in delay or obstruction in the development of cognitive skills that interweave with linguistic ability. Such children have trouble with verbal memory organization, mastery of numeracy and literacy, and higher-order cognitive processing such as executive function and theory of mind. Globally, SNHL is one of the most common among those birth conditions labeled 'defects' by the medical profession. Most deaf and hard-of-hearing children live in developing countries. In developing countries, six to seven out of 1,000 children have permanent hearing loss, most of which is SNHL. Given all of the frequency data and the trend toward speech-only training, it is clear that a significant number of children in the world with SNHL are likely to be given CIs and kept away from sign language during their early years.They run a high risk of linguistic deprivation and related cognitive deficits.

With respect to the linguistic evidence, two points can be made:

1) the recognition of the fact that both the oral-aural and the manual-visual modalities of language nourish the brain's language mechanism,

2) the recognition of changing plasticity in the brain with respect to first language acquisition.

2.1. Two modalities of language

First, language and the brain are flexible with respect to modality. Both spoken and sign languages can nurture brain development, as is shown by much research on the structure of particular spoken and sign languages and on language universals (see a multitude of articles in many linguistics journals, including Sign Language & Linguistics and Sign Language Studies, as well as more recently in journals that do not focus on sign languages, such as Language; on language processing, on neurolinguistics, on language pathologies and on second language learning. Too often in the relevant medical literature, we find the confused belief that language is equivalent to speech despite a half-century of research on sign languages. The authors recognize that absence of hearing can lead to absence of language, which can, in turn, lead to cognitive deficits, but they see 'sensory restoration'(i.e. auditory restoration) as the only way to ensure language and to prevent cognitive deficits that follow from absence of language input. This quotation is representative of the basic misconception that equates language with speech. Published policy statements about deaf children recommend early screening; early intervention; close and continued monitoring of the child's communicative, language, motor, cognitive, and social-emotional development; and protection of infant and family rights through informed choice, decision making, and consent. Frequently, such recommendations discuss almost exclusively audio-verbal therapy (AVT) via habituation and vocal output, although more recent policy statements emphasize cognitive language development and the importance of nurturing and communicating with the child regardless of modality. Nevertheless, primary care physicians express a lack of confidence in discussing follow-up procedures and intervention needs for deaf newborns because of their lack of familiarity with deafness and thus immediately refer the parents to audiologists, whose primary concern is auditory input, often with no or only skeptical recommendations of looking into sign language options. Evidence that there are at least two modalities that offer a normal pathway to language acquisition is often disregarded, leading to a failure to understand and take advantage of the flexibility of the human brain.

2.2. First language acquisition and plasticity.

The second relevant linguistic point with respect to the policy problem is that first language acquisition takes place most naturally and successfully in the first few years of life; if a child is not exposed to accessible or learnable language on a regular and frequent basis before the age of around five years old, that child is unlikely to ever use any language with native-like fluency across the grammar. Over the years we see a gradual decline in the ability to acquire a first language (note that a second language is a separate matter with distinct considerations—our concern here is first language acquisition). Some areas of the grammar seem to be resilient; that is, even in the absence of early input, they can be mastered later in life, such as word order, while other areas of language are more fragile and, without input in the very early years, tend to never get mastered, such as complex morphology, as in verb agreement. Evidence for this sensitive (or critical) period comes from children whose language development is somehow special, and from children who have been neglected and/or abused. Aphasic, bilingual, and deaf individuals reported that children with acquired aphasia can recover completely, but adults cannot, concluding that there must be a critical period for language acquisition. Later research on aphasia shows variable recovery from aphasia with children, but worse prognosis for adults. Similarly, evidence on bilingualism supports the existence of a sensitive period. In a study of twenty-year-olds comparing monolinguals, early bilinguals and late bilinguals, early bilinguals and monolinguals displayed the same level of proficiency in English and a greater proficiency than that of late bilinguals. Further, the age of onset of bilingualism was negatively correlated to English proficiency across all bilinguals. Finally, and most important to us, studies of deaf children who did not receive accessible language until after the critical period due to lack of hearing aids or because they were denied sign language , show reduced language facility. Deaf children who were first exposed to an accessible language (i.e. a sign language) at varying ages show varying degrees of mastery of language as they age, with early learners doing far better than late learners overall. Neglected and/or abused individuals. Other evidence for the first critical period comes from unfortunate incidents of neglect and abuse so severe that children did not acquire any language by the end of the first critical period and thus were linguistically deprived and accordingly severely limited in their interactions with other humans and in their cognitive functions.

The combination of these two facts, that cognitive ability can develop in either language modality or that there is a sensitive period for first language acquisition (regardless of whether abuse or neglect is involved), is of crucial relevance to the problem. Much research has shown better auditory results with earlier implantation the age of one. The problem is magnified if the child's environment is noisy and unclear. Many children do not acquire a spoken language fully with a CI, and one cannot predict with reliability which children fall into that group. The sign languages are viable human languages, with all of the cognitive benefits attributed to spoken languages. Further, sign languages are accessible to all deaf children. If deaf children acquire a sign language during the crucial period of life, they will not risk linguistic deprivation and the consequent cognitive deficits. Many studies show that deaf children trained in sign language achieve better in school than those who do not. The deaf child who acquires a sign language and then learns the written and spoken form of a spoken language is bilingual. Bilingualism has great benefits for the deaf child in cognitive, social, and educational areas.The evidence that proficiency in two or more languages results in more creative thinking in problem solving, better mental flexibility and cognitive control. All around the world children are raised multilingually, and the bilingual-bicultural trend for deaf education is a mega-trend. All deaf newborns and newly deafened small children should learn a sign language, regardless of whether they receive a hearing aid.

Several more specific recommendations follow from this basic one.

(1) Medical education must be upgraded and include linguistic thought. Medical professionals should be aware in recent research about language acquisition, specially with respect to the issues of linguistic deprivation for those children at risk, primarily hearing impaired children. Medical schools, nursing schools, and schools of public health should include this information in their syllabus.

(2) Delivery of medical care to hearing impaired children should be streamlined with the relevant health professionals, including audiologists, psychologists, surgeons, and rehabilitation teams. These teams should stay in constant contact with and respond positively to input from parents, sign language teachers, and classroom teachers. This way, the risk of linguistic deprivation can be caught timely and responded to appropriately.

(3) Recommendations from medical professionals must be precise and acceptable. Parents of deaf newborns and primarily deafened small children should be advised to teach their child sign language, in spite of whether the child also uses hearing aids or a CI. This means the entire family should learn sign language; and since the biological health of the language acquisition is at stake, this is properly a medical issue, so it is the medical profession's responsibility to counsel the parents this. When the entire family uses sign language at the dinner table, for example, the deaf child has visual access and picks up on incidental information on a variety of

topics. Developmentally, the inclusion of the child in family dialogues promotes healthy psychosocial and emotional functioning. The deaf child is likely to feel included in family conversations and is less frustrated, as is commonly reported in other situations with communication barriers. This has been self-reported as having an important impact on the deaf youth's quality of life, and the perception of being included in family dialogues is associated with fewer reports of depression symptomatology. Deaf children whose hearing parents and siblings, particularly hearing mothers, sign with them demonstrate language effectively conveying and theory of mind on a par with hearing children of the peers.

(4) More research needs to be done on second language learning, especially in a second modality. Second language learning is difficult for adults, perhaps even more so when the new language is in a different modality. Hearing relatives of a deaf child are going to need help in learning a sign language.

(5) Deaf children should be brought into contact with deaf signing children and adults frequently. The family of a deaf child should not feel the burden of being good sign language models for the child. The important point is that family members engage in frequent, direct language interaction with the deaf child, but the family must understand that their own efforts will not be enough. Parents of deaf children should help them find other deaf children to socialize with in a common language—a community of others like themselves—without continual adult intervention in that communication. Individual interpreters, who act as surrogate teachers or even parents in the classroom, often have little contact with the deaf community. As a result, deaf students can be limited to dyadic groups for communication, which do not approach the richness and complexity of language as used by a larger community. It appears the optimal way to ensure the needed exposure is to participate in group discourse. Given this, medical advisors must inform the family that the deaf child needs to be brought into contact with a community of deaf signers so as to be exposed to consistent and multiple models of signing on a regular and frequent basis. Families need to be come informed about the local culture of Deaf people and help their child (and the whole family) to participate in Deaf events.

(6) Advice from others outside the hearing sciences and medical profession must be better informed about pertinent language matters. These advisors include spiritual leaders, particularly

since the risk of depression or other psychosocial stress on the part of deaf children and their parents may bring them to these leaders for guidance. So schools of theology should include information on first language acquisition particularly as it pertains to deaf children in their curriculum.

(7) Make sign language accessible to hearing parents and their deaf child. If a family of a deaf child does not have easy access to a signing community, they must take a very strong active role in providing their child with a sign language[11].

First, the family must try to learn a sign language in the best way possible, which may require driving a substantial distance to classes. If the local community is small, the family can enlist the whole community in the effort to learn a sign language and to communicate with the deaf child in that sign language. A community might want to advertise for and hire a sign language teacher to come and stay in their community for an extended period of time, teaching everyone who is willing to learn. There are also multiple online sites and DVDs to help someone learn a sign language.

Second, the family should find out about camps for deaf children, where sign language is used and deaf children learn about and get welcomed into Deaf culture. Many such camps exist: in the United States they are scattered across the states; in Germany the German Deaf Youth Association and German Deaf Association of Hard-of-Hearing annually organize camps for Deaf and hard-of-hearing children and youth. Some have scholarships available. Some are for the entire family. There are various websites with up-to-date information on such camps (in the US: Summer Camps for Deaf and Hard of Hearing Children and Teens; 3 in Germany.

Third, the family must be resourceful. Since it is important that others sign with the deaf child, the family could start a sign language class with parents and children who are not deaf. If the family has relatives in a city with a thriving Deaf community, visiting or even arranging to spend time there may be a significant act that makes a world of difference to the child's development. The family might want to get online (using current video technology: Skype, Face Time, g Chat, Facebook, etc.) with someone who knows many people in the Deaf community to see if a Deaf family might like to come visit them for extended periods. The deaf child in one's home makes the home eligible to obtain a videophone setup from a video relay service. Alternatively, one can install videophone software in a home computer. With this setup, the family and the deaf child can talk in sign language directly via video to deaf people whom they meet and form stronger relationships. Sign language tutoring via videophone might even be arranged. These setups often cost nothing to the family except an internet connection. If the family has opportunities to live in an urban area that has a Deaf community, now might be the time to realize those opportunities. These family responsibilities can be costly in a number of ways beyond money and time. There is argument that using sign language can hinder family dynamics and that learning a sign language can be beyond the abilities of some family members, particularly older ones. We would suggest that, regardless of whether family members learn a sign language, a deaf child born into a hearing family always impacts family dynamics simply by virtue of the fact that the child is deaf. Further, every deaf child is entitled to be recognized and accepted as deaf and to develop their own identity as a deaf person.

Tthe Rights of Persons with Disabilities (2006) of the United Nations Convention emphasize to protect the rights of deaf children by 'facilitating the learning of sign language and the promotion of the linguistic identity of the deaf community' and by ensuring that their education 'is delivered in the most appropriate languages and modes and means of communication for the individual, and in environments which maximize academic and social development'. The researchers point out further that bilingual education for deaf children has not had uniform success. However, the questions of how to assure access to language in the critical years of life and how to educate deaf children are noticeably different. Many and complex educational issues arise regardless of which kind of program a child enters (whether one of the various kinds of mainstreaming programs or one of the various kinds of bilingual/bicultural programs. We are confident that present and future efforts (including more research) will lead to better-qualified teachers using more appropriate and efficacious methods and materials. The fact is that the cognitive factor that matches up best to literacy among hearing impaired children is a foundation in a first language. Much earlier work shows this, and the most recent findings continue to confirm it: those children with CIs who also sign perform better in standardized language testing than children with CIs who do not have exposure to a sign language.

(8) Government sources must fund sign language instruction for these families. Every human has a right to language. Therefore, instruction in a sign language should be funded by federal and state governments for all deaf children and their families. This funding should continue at least until the age of twelve.

(9) The current risks associated with CIs need to be reduced. The risks of harm associated with CIs should be more widely understood, and the current high risk of linguistic consequences due to using CIs only as a response to deafness in the family needs to be alleviated greatly by the use of sign language along with CIs. Cochlear implants run a host of risks beyond linguistic deprivation. All surgeries come with risks, and surgeries involving the brain may be particularly troubling. With CI surgery, many complications arise, including injury to the facial nerve, necrosis and breakdown of the flap, injury to hair follicles, improper electrode placement, post surgery infection under the flap and in the middle ear, and meningitis. There is also a huge risk (40% to 74% of patients) of vertigo that can last for years. The apparatus can fail, requiring repeated surgery with all of the same associated risks. Since many CI surgeries disable the cochlea, the implanted ear loses whatever residual hearing it had; so if the CI does not offer language access to the child, then the surgery has, in fact, had a result contrary to its very intention. The harms of cochlear implant surgery are increasing as the popularity of binaural implantation goes up, while the claimed benefits have yet to be established. Further, some deaf and hard-of-hearing children are implanted even when they already recognize up to 30% of sentence material with or without a hearing aid, which is a better recognition rate than many children have post implantation. These children actually might be losing ground with respect to speech skills. And, finally, hearing aids do not present the surgical risks of CIs and may well offer comparable or better advantages with respect to speech development, depending on the particular needs of individual children. No child should be implanted unless implantation is accompanied by sign language, and there is a very strong chance that the child will have excellent oral communication skills as a result of the child's curiosity and motivation for speaking, the child's bias toward auditory learning style, and the child's neural response to implantation.

(5)The article from https://perlinguam.journals.ac.za/pub/article/download/28/59 argues the importance of allowing hearing impaired children to acquire sign language from an age before 3 years. It demonstrates firstly that the critical/sensitive period hypothesis for language acquisition can be applied to pre-defined language aspects of spoken language as well as sign languages (i.e. aspects of formal language). This makes early diagnosis and early intervention of very crucial importance. Moreover, research findings presented in this article illustrate the advantage that sign language offers in the early years of a deaf child's life by comparing the language development landmarks of deaf learners exposed to sign language from birth to those of late-signers, orally trained deaf learners and hearing learners exposed to spoken language. The argument over the best medium of instruction for deaf learners is briefly discussed, with stress placed on the possible value of bilingual bicultural programmes to facilitate the development of deaf learners' literacy expertise.

THE CRITICAL/SENSITIVE LANGUAGE ACQUISITION HYPOTHESIS The critical period for language acquisition is the hypothesis that language is acquired best in early childhood and is more difficult to acquire later on in life. A neurologist, was one of the first scientists to propose that a lead capacity for language acquisition in children can be linked directly to the neuroplasticity of the brain in early childhood. Research on brain growth and clinical studies of brain damage, mental retardation and deafness further supported the notion of a critical period for language acquisition. In his view, successful language acquisition is limited to a period during a person's childhood years, the so-called 'window of opportunity' and extended between infancy and puberty. For some years empirical studies, both behavioural and neural, have provided further support for this hypothesis. These research results based on case studies of deaf children, isolated from first language exposure until after puberty, showed a strong relationship between the age of exposure to a language and the ultimate proficiency achieved in that language. In an attempt to counter the 'rigidity of constraints implicit in the term critical period, researchers have increasingly started to use the term sensitive periods to refer to these times between infancy and puberty' when language is learned more easily. After this sensitive period, language can be learned, but with greater difficulty and less efficiency. Although most researchers agree that a strong biological basis for language acquisition exists and that one must have appropriate experiences at the right developmental moments to acquire certain social, language, sensory and motor skills, the point in time when this critical/sensitive period ends is not well defined. According to this research the 'window of opportunity' for some visual functions extends well beyond the age of 3, until 8 or 9 years of age. Within language acquisition studies, the nature of this phenomenon has been a fiercely debated issue in psycholinguistics and cognitive science for decades. The researchers proposed that the 'window of opportunity' closes when children reach the age of 6 or 7 years, whilst other research findings suggest different sensitive periods for different language aspects. According to the researchers the sensitive periods for certain components of language such as phonology, grammatical processing and syntax occur during the fourth year of life and that for some language aspects such as semantics, it may continue even until puberty (i.e. 15 to 16 years of age).

According to one study the concept of critical / critical times for language acquisition has historically provided social policy makers a basis for the belief in initiating early intervention programs. and permanent damage that can be done if critical / critical times are not 'missed'. On the contrary, one researcher says that children's early plans can be developed without the hassle of a delicate debate over time. He challenges the view that experience should be provided between the normal ages of 0 to 3 years to ensure that children's language development continues on a regular basis. In addition, some educators are sceptical of claims that there are critical times in all forms of learning. They argue that 'critical times of hypothesis viewpoints' can reduce the acquisition of skills in reading, mathematics and other school subjects. In general, most of the research results have shown that with increasing age of language exposure there is a level of effectiveness in many language structures.

PROOF OF IMPORTANT TIME / CONFIRMATION OF SIGN LANGUAGE AVAILABLE
Sign language was specially removed from the concept of critical / critical time on the grounds that it could be successfully acquired by anyone at any age. This is a complex issue as researchers are divided on the existence of a critical / critical period for the discovery of sign language. One reason is that many deaf students have access to their primary language, sign language, at different ages and in stages of mental development; because most of them have hearing parents. This makes it difficult to compare the language acquisition stages of deaf students. According to one study, the critical period of the hypothesis has a significant impact on the overall functioning of deaf children (i.e. their language, comprehension, educational, social and emotional development) because very few hearing parents of deaf students have sign language skills. In stark contrast with the deaf children of hearing parents, deaf children with

deaf parents are given natural access and exposure to sign language from birth. As a result of signing deaf children, they perform better in all aspects of language, compared to late signatories. Two studies for deaf students (N = 71) who were indigenous or language sign language learners (acquired sign language between the ages of 9 and 16) were conducted. . Non-native signatories seem to pay more attention to identifying the structure of the voice, thus weakening their ability to recall and remember consecutive meanings. In contrast, traditional signatories analyze lexical structure automatically, better understand and make different types of artistic changes. These findings suggest that sign language was not as easy to learn as it had been initially suggested by some researchers, as well as demonstrating the advanced skills of indigenous sign language scientists. Focusing on the critical / critical times of sign language discovery, the findings of the study suggest that there may be a natural basis for the development of sign language. In these studies Deep deaf children with no sign language or language (other than their parents' language) developed sign language communication programs such as many official spoken languages.

Some researchers say that critical times can be determined separately (i.e. by external factors) and the basic biological process. In addition, research has shown that deaf students with hearing-impaired parents who are able to sign language may have the same language as hearing students and, in some cases, even younger students. Since most deaf students are born into deaf families, many researchers emphasize the importance of early detection and hearing aids as important factors in ensuring proper language acquisition at a critical time in language development. According to another study, deaf students should be diagnosed as soon as possible, preferably immediately after birth; and the intervention should take place before the child is six months old so that the deaf students can experience the same stages of development as hearing students. The findings of the study provide further support in the critical period of sign language acquisition. As with spoken languages, there has been a marked difference in language between those who learn sign language as native speakers (from birth) and those who learn it later. Indigenous signatories are able to apply morphological 1 sign language features in more appropriate situations than late signatories. In addition, indigenous scientists use a number of local languages and are able to change the grammar and syntax of their native language. In other research, deaf participants tend to make logical or spurious mistakes, compared to phonetic errors that were directly related to age when they first learned American sign language. which means that as the age of adoption increased there was a corresponding increase in facial-related errors, phonetic incentives). In addition, as discussed in this paper, the importance of providing deaf students with adequate language acquisition at an early age is beneficial to the language development of deaf students, as well as their mental and emotional well-being. To further clarify this concept we will compare the language acquisition stages of deaf learners who use spoken language with those who communicate with sign language in the next section. History of language acquisition for deaf learners: spoken language compared to sign language To hear children learn the language of their native language through contact and communication with spoken language. At a critical juncture in listening and language preparation, they develop the ability to distinguish between sounds and words, and begin to assign meaning to words. At six to eight months, hearing children begin to understand simple language, and at the age of one, they begin to utter simple words. About five years old they begin to understand the syntax of spoken language. A deaf child growing up with hearing parents experiences the development of a spoken language in a completely different way. Deaf students who speak a language raised in a spoken language face a very difficult challenge to understand that unintelligible lip movements some people actually represent. In addition, they are expected to give meaning to the spoken language and to learn to speak it. Contrary to their hearing-impaired peers, the discovery of spoken language provides few language effects for deaf students. Some research results show that hearing three-year-old participants have a vocabulary of spoken language between 1000 and 2000 words, and five-year-old adult language participants receive vocabulary in their study. spoken less than 29 words. In addition, research results show that deaf learners find it extremely difficult to acquire spoken language and that their listening and descriptive language skills are directly impaired by the acquisition of spoken language. During a 15-month-long intervention, a 30-month-old deaf child was able to learn only one word a month. In contrast, most hearing students (aged 30 to 48 months) can automatically read 60 to 120 words a month. In the study the comprehension of spoken vocabulary among the deaf participants (ages 8 to 12) was significantly lower than expected for a four-year-old deaf child, while the comprehension skills of eight-year-old Canadian deaf students were similar to those for four-year-old children.

Letters   from
https://www.researchgate.net/publication/309430437_THE_BENEFITS_OF_SIGN_LANGUAG
E_FOR_DEAF_LEARNERS_WITH_LANGUAGE_CHALLENGES show that most people
with hearing (over 70 dB) are fluent in speech. especially in situations that require the delivery of
simple messages, where there are indications of a 'rich' context. However, there are many
relevant issues regarding concepts such as rhyme, breathing, phoning, vocalization, especially
speech. Less than 20% of the speech of deaf people is easily recognizable or audible to the
average listener. Clearly, the acquisition of spoken language is a very difficult and difficult task
for many deaf students. In addition, it seems that the acquisition of spoken language does not
guarantee adequate communication opportunities for the deaf, and it also contributes to the
limited access to their language. This raises the question of whether it would be better for deaf
learners to be exposed to sign language as a natural / first language during language sensitivity.
Sign language The results of this study provide a strong argument that sign language acquisition
can have an unparalleled value for deaf students. Researchers argue that most deaf students have
the ability to learn sign language as a natural language. Deaf students who are exposed to sign
language by their deaf parents from birth begin to applaud (with their hands) before making their
first signs. The sign-language section for deaf students is an essential element in the construction
of sign language. At this stage, deaf children begin to associate their sign names with visual
signal patterns - hence, the sign propagation phase gradually changes into a single 'word' (sign)
category, then a 'word' (sign) category, and eventually found There is a 'continuation between
phonetics and vocabulary forms used in deaf infants and their first signs' and reports that the
most common places and hand gestures were observed in the bible and were most common at the
first signs of deaf children. It seems that most researchers are of the opinion that deaf students
acquire sign language in the same way that hearing-impaired students acquire a spoken language,
but there appear to be differences of opinion on the age of the acquisition of deaf students. Some
researchers argue that deaf children get their first symptoms before students of the world get
their first names. One researcher takes a different view; that these researchers mistakenly
interpreted the whispering category of deaf children as 'early symptoms'. Another undeniable
feature is that hearing children also interact with signals during the buzz phase. One report points
to striking similarities in the use of sign language for deaf and hearing impaired children in pre-
language (nine to 12 months) and post-language (12 to 48 months) language acquisitions.

On the contrary, recent findings confirm the work of previous researchers. Compared with research studies showing that most hearing children with normal language development begin to utter their first names at about 13 months, deaf children in one study produced early symptoms (eight months old). In addition, the researcher questioned the results of the study on the grounds that the validity and validity of these results were limited by the small sample size in the study. Their research results showed that when deaf students found sign language in a natural environment, it was acquired in the same way that hearing students found spoken language. The study focused not only on the number of words (symbols) of deaf students in certain ages, but also on the content of these words. up to 23 productive vocabulary (symbols or words) of deaf learners and students who hear it compares very well and is almost identical. The study reveals very strong similarities between the first dictionary content for hearing and hearing students. The use of nouns, especially the names of people, animals and food, is very similar. It is also noteworthy that hearing students compose animal sounds, and animal sounds are not part of the vocabulary of deaf students. In addition, the results of a study conducted in a South African study of deaf (N = 60) students in a rural area in the Free State, showed that reading and spelling skills of deaf students could be significantly improved by exposing these students, although this study did not compare the language movements of deaf learners. of hands, these research results have strengthened the positive impact of early literacy interventions for deaf students at a time when so-called critical language acquisition. and the importance of SASL to help develop the skills of English-speaking illiterate students. In addition, some of the findings of the study also show that sign language skills are closely related to English literacy skills. 'between sign language and English literacy d development. The concept of multilingualism 'states that all languages share the same basic skills and that the cognitive and learning skills acquired in the first language will transmit skills related to the second language. The first 35 words (English) and signals for the deaf and the deaf respectively.

(6) The reason for choosing sign language as the language of communication and the language of instruction for deaf learners There is no denying the importance of language acquisition in the general performance of deaf learners. That is obvious. However, any language that should be considered the first / native language of deaf learners in the school environment continues to be challenged. Decisions made in the language of communication and the language of instruction

directly affect the ability of deaf learners to master the language and influence the choice of strategies used to teach these students. The three teaching methods that have received the most support are the oral (oral) method, complete communication and sign language. The oral reading approach is said to build their reading skills through a 'phonological pathway' (a pathway to literacy based on phonological analysis). This method involves the training of hearing, speaking and lip reading and prevents signing or gestures of any kind. In oral teaching the main purpose of 'getting used' by deaf learners is to adapt better to the hearing world by making them more verbal. By responding to the oral tradition, there was a breakthrough in the perfect way to communicate in the 1970's. As a philosophy, this approach encourages teachers to communicate with their deaf students using simultaneous communication methods (speaking, English, sign language, gestures and speech learning) - this is called Signed Support English. Because of its emphasis on spoken language, many deaf students face difficulties with the overall communication process because the dictionary and the structure of the bilingual grammar (signed and spoken English) are different. Deaf students do not seem to be able to process and sign fluently at the same time. The need for a deaf child to learn to deal with deaf and dumb culture has made it possible to speak bilingual programs. Bilingualism in South Africa means that South African Sign Language (SASL) is introduced as a first language as early as possible, and that native language (English) is acquired as a second language. written on it.

RESULTS OF SOUTH AFRICAN SIGN LANGUAGE TEACHING

South Africa's position on the provision of learners with barriers to learning and development (including deaf students) is clearly stated in the provisions of the Special Needs Draft Bill: In adopting this inclusive approach we acknowledge that the most vulnerable students in South Africa are barred by those with special needs. much has been made possible due to the history and level of academic support provided. While providing a decent educational environment in which deaf students thrive is an ongoing concern for policy makers and academics alike, it remains a serious problem. Some researchers / educators adopt the 'inclusion philosophy'. They argue that inclusive education works better than segregated education because it eliminates the prejudices and questionable conduct associated with special schools. While support for mainstreaming (globally) support in special education generally (based on ethical, educational and economic factors), however, many educators say there is ample evidence of failure of standard programs for deaf children. Trainers and therapists, inaccessible places, etc. Given South Africa's history of language education policies (based on apartheid ideology), issues related to human rights with regard to education, language and culture have been a major concern for the South African government in the post-apartheid era. It is beyond the scope of this article to discuss in detail the South African language policies, but the authors would like to point out that much work has been done at the policy level to protect and develop the 11 official languages (including SASL). Although SASL is not one of the official languages, it is addressed directly to the South African Constitution and other related policy documents. According to them, the dictionary project overemphasized group-based diversity, with some feeling that the emphasis on a single SASL program would degrade the languages of the deaf. Despite the progress made in promoting and establishing SASL as a first / natural language for deaf people, in fact, many deaf students are not taught through SASL, as many Deaf Teachers' teachers cannot sign and still believe that deaf children should learn the local language. The researcher states that 'it is in this way that deaf students are disabled: teachers and the language-blind system which is their basic human right (i.e. SASL), and without them they have no real access to learning'. In addition, Deaf educators still do not need to have formal training and / or degrees in Deaf Education. As a result many hearing teachers in these schools have little or no knowledge of the effects of learning on teaching literacy (either oral or in sign language instructions). They strongly opposed the inclusion of deaf students in Special Schools. To highlight the fact that many deaf students, despite being placed in deaf schools, are still excluded from equal opportunities and equal education. This 'paradox' has a significant impact on the academic success of deaf learners because the literacy results of deaf learners are much lower than those of hearing students: most of them work below Grade 4 when they leave school. in order to create a barrier and supportive learning environment for deaf students there are many implications for one to consider. CONCLUSION / RECOMMENDATIONS

A literature review of this study highlights the importance of early diagnosis and intervention for two important reasons. Firstly, important research results show that the critical time of language acquisition can also be applied to the acquisition of sign language. Second, deaf students with deaf parents who have been exposed to sign language from birth are more likely to acquire successive language classes as hearing students and, in some cases, even younger than hearing students. In contrast, the discovery of 'late' language negatively affects the language skills of deaf learners, as well as their social and emotional development. Factors that directly affect this include their grammar, language processing and cognitive skills. The acquisition of spoken language seems to offer very little opportunities for communication for deaf students. A detailed comparison of the language acquisition measures for deaf learners with sign language and those taught in spoken language shows the immeasurable importance of sign language for deaf learners. For this reason, along with the possible loss of ownership, an inclusive education for all deaf students in South Africa is a controversial area. The education system as a whole should find solutions tailored to the characteristics of deaf learners 'which will help them to develop not only linguistically but also emotionally, socially and academically'. In conclusion, we would like to make the following recommendations / comments: Early detection of hearing loss (identification), early access to the education system • and early contact with signers are key to ensuring that deaf students can and learn the language Early intervention services, including family listening support and parental training sessions to improve their sign language skills, can prevent or significantly reduce communication, social and emotional barriers and development resulting from hearing loss. , other. The Institute for the Deaf Education, South Africa, has launched an early intervention program. Through this program parent counsellors (impartially) assist parents in making decisions about their children's language development, communication and other issues related to learning, learning, play and general developmental issues and help to achieve selected parents. Deaf people in South Africa are properly trained, have sufficient knowledge of deaf education and must be bilingual in SASL and spoken (written) language (eg English). , a concerted effort should be made to encourage deaf students to become teachers in order to educate the many deaf students in schools for the deaf; Recognizing that many teachers are currently unable to sign, the emphasis during the 'interim phase', should be on pre-service training and on-the-job training and recruitment of deaf adults (e.g. exemplars and teaching assistants) in school classrooms. (7)Introduction

In areas with a large Deaf community, almost everyone knows or has met someone who is Deaf or Hard of Hearing (D/HH) but very few people understand the obstacles that deaf or hard of hearing persons face. Deaf individuals have severe hearing loss and hard of hearing individuals have hearing loss that falls on a spectrum from mild to profound. Typically, deaf students are academically behind their hearing peers and mathematics is one of the areas where they face learning challenges. For example, if a deaf student goes to a public state or local school for the deaf the teacher may be fluent in American Sign Language (ASL) but may lack pedagogical content knowledge (PCK) of how to teach mathematical concepts for understanding. Also, a deaf student could be mainstreamed in a mathematics class with an excellent teacher but have an interpreter that cannot communicate the mathematics being taught effectively. Such common communication challenges may begin to explain why the deaf or hard of hearing students are academically behind their hearing peers. It is well known that mathematical concepts become more abstract and harder to comprehend in middle and high school, and for deaf individuals the language barrier may be a factor that makes this abstraction even more difficult. For the remainder of this paper, DHH will be used to refer to the population of Deaf and Hard of Hearing students. List of Terms To guide the reader through the content in this work, the following terms are defined: Deafness – Defined by the Individuals with Disabilities Education Act (IDEA), it is a hearing impairment that is so severe that the child is impaired in processing linguistic information through hearing, with or without amplification. Deafness falls on the extreme end of the spectrum as severe.

Hard of hearing – A hearing impairment that falls between mild and profound on the spectrum Deaf culture – A set of social beliefs, behaviors, art, literary traditions, history, values, and shared institutions of communities that are influenced by deafness and which use sign languages as the main means of communication. When used as a cultural label especially within the culture, the word deaf is often written with a capital D and referred to as "big D Deaf" in speech and sign. When used as a label for the audiological condition, it is written with a lower case d. For example: "He is Deaf", means that he is a member of the Deaf Community while "He is deaf" means that he is lacking the sense of hearing. Residential schools – An institution where students typically go and live full time or during the week while attending school. These can be private or state schools. All the students in the school are deaf or hard of hearing. They are often educated by deaf teachers or teachers who are trained in deafness. Some residential schools offer day-only options for students that are able to commute from home.

Conceptual Understanding – Demonstrated by recognizing, labeling, and generating examples of concepts; using and interrelating models, diagrams, manipulatives, and representations of concepts, identifying and applying principles, comparing and contrasting, and integrating relating concepts and principles Procedural Fluency - the ability to apply procedures accurately, efficiently, and flexibly; transfer procedures to different problems and contexts; to build or modify procedures from other procedures; and to recognize when one strategy or procedure is more appropriate to apply than another.

Mathematical Reasoning – The ability to think logically about the relationships among DEAF STUDENTS IN MATHEMATICS

Such reasoning is valid and stems from careful consideration of alternatives, and includes knowledge of how to justify conclusions. Pedagogical Content Knowledge - The overlap of information about subject knowledge, that is knowledge of the subject being taught, and the knowledge of how to teach. It includes an understanding of what makes the learning of specific topics easy or difficult: the conceptions and preconceptions that students of different ages and backgrounds bring with them to learning.

 Knowledge of Content and Students – the intertwining of a teacher's knowledge of subject content and their students, it is the understanding of how the students will interact with the content.

Performance Gap – Students classified as hearing impaired are generally 2 years behind their hearing peers. As the students progress, the performance gap grows. Common Core State Standards (CCSS) – A set of academic standards in mathematics and English that were created to ensure that all students graduate from high school with the necessary skills and knowledge to succeed in the future.

Analysis of Variance (ANOVA) – A statistical method used to analyze areas of significant differences among group means. It provides a test of whether or not the means of several groups are equal.

Research in the field of deafness and deaf culture show that DHH students are approximately two years behind their hearing equivalents. Specifically, in mathematics, DHH students graduate at a fifth or sixth grade comprehension level. The research done by many has targeted specific mathematical topics that are typically the most difficult. These topics include problem solving, measurements, estimation, patterns, and more. However, this data only looks at young DHH children and because the majority of deaf studies include pre-kindergarten through second grade (ages 3 to 8), there is a great lack of information for DHH students past the eighth grade. It could be assumed that the performance gap for DHH pre-kindergarten and kindergarten children extends to DHH high school students. Previous research leads into an examination of the widening performance gap for DHH in high school mathematics. The performance gap is approximately two years and seemingly continues to grow as students continue through high school. It is not clear if the performance gap centers on problem solving specifics such as conceptual understanding, procedural fluency, and mathematical reasoning. Thus, the purpose of this research is to determine how conceptual understanding, procedural fluency, and mathematical reasoning contribute to DHH students' learning of mathematics in comparison to their hearing peers.

Literature Review Research provides a background on mathematics performance for both hearing and DHH students. The students without hearing loss in fourth and eighth grade show increasing average mathematics scores. Half of those DHH students fell below a third and fifth grade level respectively. In problem solving, similar results were reported. For fourth graders, 80% scored average or below average, with half scoring just above a second grade level. For eighth graders, 80% scored average or below and half of eighth graders at only a fourth grade level (Pagliaro, 2006). Many researchers in the field of deaf studies are concerned with why and when the performance gap begins. It is known that about 50% of DHH students have a co-occurring disability. Some professionals may be hesitant to diagnose other disabilities in a student who is DHH because of the difficulty in ruling out the student's hearing loss and reduced exposure to language and communication models as a primary cause of a disability. However, ruling out any co-occurring disabilities, there is no difference in cognitive abilities between deaf and hearing students. Instead, it is possibly the language barrier, experiences, and instruction in a child's life that play a role in their mathematics performance. Humans incidentally learn mathematical concepts at a young age. For example, a parent may count toes or use words like "big" or "little" to identify a sibling. Mathematical concepts, like quantity, develop from infancy and children begin to mathematize between ages 3 and 6. Children intuitively develop concepts from numbers to geometry.DHH children most often lack those experiences and parental instruction because of the language barrier assuming the parents do not sign. DHH children who know American Sign Language (ASL) show average or better skills in object counting. These children understood a one-to-one correspondence between object and sign. They chose to study familiarity, imagery, signability, and concreteness. Of the four factors, imagery proved to be the best predictor of term recall. This supports research that argues that terms represented by a single sign are recalled well than terms represented by compound signs. But, further research on other mathematical concepts did not show similar results. Young DHH children scored average or below average in many other categories, especially story problems, also known as word or applied problems. At any age or grade level, story problems tend to be a large part of mathematics and classroom instruction. Typically, an individual without DHH can pick up necessary vocabulary as well as numbers to correctly solve the problem, but this is more of a challenge for DHH students. A study done on young DHH children examined their ability to solve word problems. Another researcher found that the children did not connect the story language to arithmetic functions important in solving the problem. Even when the story was presented in ASL the children did not view the story as having any links to the numbers. In general, the children were missing the linguistic cues that would make the problem easier to solve. Pedagogical Best Practices The discussions of the pedagogical best practices are not unique for the field of DHH education. There is framework surrounding what pedagogical content knowledge (PCK) is and how it relates to students' mathematical outcomes. The research leads to an examination and conceptualization of teachers' knowledge of content and students (KCS). Both PCK and KCS are argued to be crucial in a classroom, for both DHH and hearing students. KCS is defined as "content knowledge intertwined with knowledge of how students think about, know, or learn this particular content". Using pedagogical content knowledge best practices can have a tremendous affect on student performance.

(8) The research relates to young people aged 0 – 25, with specific empirical focus on young people aged 16 – 25. Through in-depth interviews and online surveys, the research engaged with 20 disabled and D/deaf young people across Scotland, alongside a number of individuals working within the Scottish youth arts sector and in disability and D/deaf arts.

The research find that young disabled and deaf people face multiple and intersecting barriers to accessing arts provision. Five main barriers were identified:

1. Finding suitable arts provision;

2. Availability of access information;

3. Lack of provision for access and support;

4. Travel, transport and location; and

5. Attitudes and awareness of arts providers.

The research identified five key strategies to address these barriers:

1. Provision specifically for young disabled and D/deaf people;

2. Centralised information about arts opportunities;

3. Front Door to Stage Door Access provision;

4. Connections built with disabled and D/deaf communities across Scotland; and

5. Education and awareness for arts providers.

These strategies offer arts providers concrete recommendations for improving disabled and D/deaf access. It is anticipated that, in light of this report, organisations and agencies providing arts opportunities to young people will be better informed of the barriers faced by young disabled and D/deaf people, and better equipped to address these barriers and improve access to their provision. This report outlines research conducted to investigate the barriers faced by disabled and D/deaf young people in accessing youth arts provision.

The purpose of this research was to identify the main barriers faced by young disabled and D/deaf people in accessing arts provision, in order to enable arts providers to be better informed of the barriers faced by this group of young people. The barriers were identified through conducting interviews and surveys with young disabled and D/deaf people, alongside exchanges with individuals working within the youth arts sectors. The research investigated what arts providers can do to improve access to provision, in order to develop solid recommendations for arts providers to utilise when considering disabled and D/deaf access. Again, these recommendations have been directly shaped and informed by the empirical research conducted with young disabled and D/deaf people.

Why is this research area important? This research area is important because it addresses a major lacuna in arts scenes: the dearth of disabled and D/deaf people on stages and screens, in front of and behind television cameras, in the books we read and the films we watch, on governing bodies and in management positions, and at the front of classrooms delivering arts provision to future generations of artists. It is imperative to understand the barriers faced by young special and hearing impaired human beings.in order to equip arts providers with the knowledge of how to better enable access and thus nurture the next generation of disabled and D/deaf talent. The purpose of this research was to instigate a meaningful dialogue with young disabled and D/deaf people and, through this report, with arts providers. While previous empirical research has been conducted into young disabled and D/deaf artists1, no such research has explored across artforms the specific barriers faced by young disabled and hearing impaired in accessing youth arts provision in Scotland. It is anticipated that, in light of the findings from this research, arts providers will be better informed of the barriers to access faced by young disabled and D/deaf people. Moreover, this report aims to establish tangible and practical recommendations to enable arts providers to improve access for young disabled and D/deaf people. Defining the research terms to provide context and clarity, briefly outlined and defined below are the main terms used within the research. Arts: The research employs a cross-artform definition of the arts, incorporating: • Performance-based arts, such as drama, dance and physical theatre;• Writing, such as creative writing, scriptwriting, and arts-related journalism. Disabled: The research employs the social model of disability to frame and define the terms 'disabled' and 'disability', wherein people are disabled by society and barriers are created by external socio-cultural structures and the physical environment. This marks a shift away from the medical model, which places onus on an individual's impairments as the source of barriers. When employing this term, self-identification is key. D / Deaf: Research uses the term 'D / deaf' to integrate the plural and cultural diversity of D / deaf communities. The term refers to people and communities who are deaf, deaf, hard of hearing and hearing impaired. For many people, the Deaf (italics 'D') identifies a different identity, culture and language - the British Sign Language (BSL). Often, the Deaf are considered to be separate from the disabled. However, much like the social model of disability, D/deaf people too face barriers within mainstream hearing-centric culture and society. Again, when employing these terms, self-identification is key.

Research Questions

The three main Research Questions for the research were as follows:

1. What arts activities are young disabled and D/deaf people currently engaging in?

2. What barriers are faced by young disabled and D/deaf people in accessing arts provision?

3. What factors would improve young disabled and D/deaf people's access to youth arts provision?

Research Design: This research used an inductive approach and qualitative design, utilising both in-depth semi-structured interviews and an online survey.

The purpose of the research design was to instigate a dialogue with young people about their experiences of participating in the arts as disabled and D/deaf people. The data from the empirical research was analyses manually, utilising a 'grounded theory' approach. Interview Design: The interviews utilised a semi-structured design, consisting of a series of questions and topics drawn directly from the Research Questions. Interviews were conducted face to-face and over the telephone, depending upon the method most suitable to the individual young person. Face-to-face interviews typically took place in public locations (such as cafés) as suggested by participants. The duration of interviews was typically between 45 minutes and 1 hour, per interview. Interviews were conducted verbally and/or via a BSL interpreter. Interactive interview materials were made available to stimulate topic-specific conversation, using the Spectral Elicitation method.

Survey Design: The online survey was created on Google Forms and launched during November 2015. Two versions of the survey were made: a main version and an Easy Read version. The surveys were tested to ensure they were compatible with screen-reading and online text-to-speech software (ChromeVox). The purpose of the survey was twofold: firstly, to recruit interview participants through promoting the research and acquainting prospective participants with the research; and secondly, to provide an alternative to participating in an interview.

The first page of the survey fully briefed prospective participants about the research. The survey questions consisted of:

• Demographic questions, e.g. age, location, disability and D/deaf identity.

• Which artforms are you interested in? (Multiple choice) Drama and theatre; Dance and physical theatre; Music; Visual arts; Film; Other (please state).

• Do you take part in any groups or activities? (Paragraph answer)

• What difficulties or barriers have you faced in getting involved in the arts? (Paragraph answer)
• Questions relating to interview participation and usage of personal information.

Participation criteria: The criteria for participating in the empirical research were that the young people

1. Were aged between 0 and 25;

2. self-identified as disabled and/or as D/deaf;

3. Were involved in or wanted to be involved in the arts; and

4. Currently resided in Scotland.

(9)Sample Size: A total of 20 young people participated in the empirical research, including 7 young people who participated in in-depth qualitative interviews. Age: The average age of those participating in the research was 22, with most participants being aged between 18 and 25 years.

Range of Disabilities: The majority of the participants in the research identified as disabled. In addition to disability, four participants identified as D/deaf or as both D/deaf and disabled.

FINDINGS For the young people with less-visible or invisible disabilities and for the young D/deaf people, they often encountered assumptions that equated age and youth with being non D/deaf and non-disabled. These young people discussed how they often faced expectations to perform tasks that were incompatible with their physical, mental, or linguistic capabilities. Meanwhile, the young people with more visible disabilities tended to encounter assumptions that underestimated or overlooked their capacities and autonomy. Artistic Practice and Worth: Attitudes towards disabled and D/deaf people's artistic practice and worth emerged as a barrier, with some young people discussing how their artistic practice and worth is viewed differently by others as a result of being disabled or D/deaf. These young people discussed how they as individuals and their artistic work can be viewed as tragic or inspirational. Some of these young people also discussed how narratives around disability often follow a set script or pattern of 'overcoming adversity', often produced for the purpose of 'inspiring' non-disabled people. In addition to this, some of the young people discussed how they feel limited by the expectation to make work only about being disabled or D/deaf.

Awareness of Disabled and D/deaf Issues, Identities and Access: The young people also discussed the impact of arts providers' awareness of both issues pertaining to disabled and D/deaf people and disabled and D/deaf access as barriers to accessing provision. The young people stated that arts providers' awareness of disabled and D/deaf issues and of access considerations is vital to ensuring provision is accessible to them. The young people offered many practical recommendations to aid arts providers' awareness of disabled and D/deaf issues and access, which are discussed in the next section.

Some of the young people currently attended or had attended Special Educational Needs schools and schools with specialist D/deaf units and visual impairment units. While these young people had positive experiences of engaging in arts provision in these school settings, once they left formal education they faced barriers in locating suitable arts provision. Such scenarios present real challenges to young people who wish to continue engaging in the arts.

Given the specific barriers discussed throughout this report and the experiences shared by the young people, it may be beneficial for youth arts providers to consider building connections with: • Special Educational Needs schools/education units; • D/deaf schools/education units and community groups; • Blind and visual impairment schools/education units; • Young people in areas of socio-economic deprivation; • Young people in rural or less populated areas.

CONCLUDING STATEMENT The findings discussed throughout this report suggest that young disabled and D/deaf people face multiple and intersecting barriers to accessing youth arts provision. While working within acknowledged limitations, this research has identified the barriers to access and offered concrete recommendations for how access to arts provision might be improved for disabled and D/deaf young people.Common misconceptions Most deaf people and their culture are a mystery to those in the hearing world. Lack of hearing aids for deaf people has led to certain misconceptions about the deaf community as evidenced by the following take from the Metro Regional Service Center for Deaf and Hard of Hearing People: All Deaf people want to hear , many are proud to be part of the Deaf Community and enjoy the rich art of the Deaf Culture. They do not view this as a disability or a hindrance. Most deaf people have deaf parents In fact, less than 5% of deaf children have deaf parents. More than 90% of deaf parents have hearing children and 90% of deaf children were born to hearing parents. All Deaf People Are Silent This common misconception is based on the sensible choices made by deaf people not to use their voice. Actually some Deaf people speak and they do well. Many of those who do not use their voice choose not to use it for many reasons. Some believe that others will not understand them or that their volume will be too high for some settings. All deaf people can read Lips while most deaf people may be able to read other people's lips; many choose not to learn this craft. In fact, only 30% of English language can be seen on the lips, because most words have the same movement of the outer lip and differ only in the direction of the inner mouth. Most people who prefer lip reading are harder to hear than completely deaf; because they can distinguish some sounds to read lips is easy. All Deaf People Use Sign Language While many prefer to use American Sign Language or some other sign system; others prefer alternative communication methods. Some who lose their hearing later in life do not use sign language. Deaf People Lead a Different Life to Hearing People

In fact, deaf people are living similar lives to hearing people. They drive, get married, have children, go to school or work, go to markets or shopping malls, and pay their bills. Some differences exist, such as where they go to school or how they use the telephone. Deaf People Can Not Use the Phone In fact, new technologies has led to the development of deaf devices, including those that allow them to use their phones. Many deaf families have a special ringer with a flashing light to indicate when the phone is ringing. Once on the phone, many have created video chat channels where two deaf people can see and sign. They also have the ability to communicate with hearing people using TTYs / TDDs (typewriters) connected directly to telephone lines. Or they can use a new device: video translators. Deaf People Who Cannot Enjoy Movies or Music What about Beethoven? He was deaf and became one of the greatest composers in the world. Deaf people "hear" vibrations in music rather than "hear" them, as their peers do.

Also, there are deaf dancers, artists, actors, and complete deaf theatre companies. In movie theatres or DVDs there is an option to add captions or other audio / visual tools to help them. All Deaf People Use Hearing aids although many people benefit from the use of hearing aids because of their ability to amplify loud noises such as alarms or sirens, which can allow them to avoid potential accidents or accidents, many do not benefit at all. In fact, the use of hearing aids depends on a number of factors depending on the individual. Hearing Ears Restore Hearing "Hearing aids amplify sound, but do not adjust the hearing. They have no effect on a person's ability to process that sound. In cases where hearing loss interferes with incoming sounds, hearing aids can do nothing to correct it. In fact, it can make the distraction worse. A hearing aid can make a person hear a person's voice, but they can understand different words". All Deaf people are not so smart

"Deafness does not affect indigenous intelligence or the body's ability to produce sounds." When a person hears or does not say this, in any way, it does not mean that he cannot read and acquire knowledge. Language Acquisition "A major educational challenge for deaf learners is finding the language of their native language and not just the production of speech but also the language system itself. For many learners the language of the community is not their first language, in the sense that they may not be able to master the same language as the native language, or, traditionally, the second language, in the sense that they may be exposed at an early age in any other language. "Language Learning Area for Deaf Learners: In all cultures, language is a major unifying factor. From birth, a baby begins to learn the language of the house. In Spanish, English, or American Sign Language, a child learns to communicate with his parents. Although there are many stages of this process of learning the steps do not differ much between spoken languages. Children living in families with different levels of textbooks and whose parents speak and read are more likely to succeed in school. Conversely, when children do not have access to the same material as their classmates and their parents do not participate in discussions or emphasize the importance of reading and writing, they often do wrong

The school is, although there is a difference: A child who grew up in a rich home with books and interviewed parents is more likely to succeed in school than a child who grew up in a home without books or interviews. Although both children have the same ability to read, it shows that "care" is an important part of education.

Status of Early Language Acquisition for Deaf Children: 1) Children whose parents are deaf and who use American Sign Language as their primary means of communication in daily life. 2) Children with hearing or deaf parents who use a combination of American Sign Language and spoken English in everyday life. 3) Children with hearing parents use only spoken language. Many people think that deaf children have parents who are deaf; however, only 5% of deaf children come from deaf parents.

One deaf signator explained his study plan as follows: "

1) Read the article several times, 2) Write notes, 3) Write non-grammar, ie BSL, 4) Then write in English, 5) Talk to someone, 6) Final draft of the article (takes 3 Although British Sign Language is very different In American Sign Language the meaning of this quote is the same. The process that deaf students go through is much more time consuming than their hearing partners. many deaf students learning English are similar to those of foreign English students as a second language, and the songs written for deaf students and ESL at the same level of proficiency seem to be the same above all else ".Conclusion: There is a great need to change the way deaf students learn English. The much-needed change is due to the number of deaf students entering colleges and universities without proper foundations. Changes must be made to the first

and / or second level or the cycle will continue. These changes should include: including ASL and English in all subjects, having an assessment strategy for oral and written communication, and the time devoted to the basics of written English and how it differs from the "spoken" in which most people learn to write. This method, although partially installed in some schools across the country, is not fully implemented. This seems to be the best way to teach deaf students the latest trends and the great support of two ASL and English immersion schools. While this process, as a whole, is still part of its ideas that have been shown to be effective, such as Oregon School for the Deaf. However, further research needs to be done in relation to the writing of deaf students included in the course for a few generations. Perhaps we should examine the enrolment of deaf students from the 1980's and compare it to that of current students, to see the changes made at a large and small scale. This will prove or disprove the advantages of both teaching methods compared to other methods such as the "Total Communication Method".

(10) ABSTRACT This article is based on a qualitative case study of teachers' conceptions of improvisation in teaching. We can identify four specific characteristics of how improvisation in teaching is conceived; improvisation of design, improvisation in communication, and improvisation dependent on repertoire and context.

Our research question is: What kinds of conceptions of improvisation as a professional teaching skill can be identified in in-service MA students' research-based descriptions and reflections on teaching? Based on our findings, we shall discuss the implications for the teacher's role and for teacher education.

Improvisus is a Latin word, which means 'the unforeseen'. To improvise is to be open to new perspectives and actions, with an expectation for what is not yet, but which can be realised.We often think of improvisation as an everyday activity, i.e. intuitive and spontaneous actions in a challenging situation. Improvisational practices in the music and theatre traditions have strongly influenced educational theory and practice.

In the field of education, improvisation is often seen as an applied, specific teaching tool or skill developed in the profession of teaching where it can be learned and rehearsed. However, several researchers underline the importance of having a broad approach to our understanding of improvisation, arguing that improvisation is interwoven in everyday life. Improvisation as a teaching skill In education, there is no common understanding or definition of a teaching skill.. The teacher must meet the students with respect and integrity, a meeting that represents an asymmetrical power relation. escriptions of improvisation in teaching vary from the ability to make spontaneous decisions and solve problems, there and then, to the enactment of concrete instructions regarding what to do. This means that teachers' conceptions and practice of improvisation must be related to discussions about value-based instructions regarding what to do in school and about curriculum contents and teaching skills. A skill can be defined as the mastering of a concrete problem, e.g. in mathematics, or more generally as developing new literacy competences. Teachers must improvise to handle challenges in the twenty-first century, with a focus on creativity, critical thinking, innovation and problem-solving, underlining students as active participants and co-constructors of knowledge.

Four dimensions or aspects of improvisation: 1) structure and design: a dimension characterised by teachers' handling, altering and carrying out sequences of lessons on the basis of spontaneous input from students or contexts; 2) communication and dialogues: a dimension characterised by how teachers develop and carry out learning-focused dialogue with students on the basis of spontaneous input; 3) repertoire: a dimension characterised by teachers making contextual and learning-focused choices of examples and activities in lessons on the basis of their professional subject-oriented and didactical knowledge/orientation and 4) context: a dimension characterised by teachers establishing an improvisational practice in a certain domain, theme or context.

Research findings: Our findings suggest that disciplined improvisation should be seen as a professional teaching skill. Thus, it has to be integrated in student teachers' knowledge base and form part of the discussion regarding their responsibility, accountability and autonomy. Given that improvisation is not addressed in the current steering documents schools or teacher education, we might ask whether, and how, student teachers can develop professional improvisational competences or skills. This implies that improvisation needs to be added to the agenda as collaboration between student teachers, teacher educators and practicum teachers, not only as a theoretical theme, but also with practices in different situations and at different levels. There is, however, no explicit focus on improvisation in the new steering documents, and we find it highly relevant to seek a discussion about the potential of improvisation in the teacher education reform (in terms of didactics, subject knowledge, interaction and collaboration, rehearsal and research).Experienced teachers and teacher educators have to collaborate with student teachers to combine practice and theoretical reflections. Student teachers must thus get the chance to observe, explore and try out improvisational practice in an environment they trust. In teacher education, one has to develop a toolbox and train in and reflect on improvisation. We argue that such reflections are a hallmark of becoming a professional, improvising teacher. However, the vignette presented in the introduction illustrates that improvising is risky. We may thus ask whether teachers and student teachers simply move from an 'instructional ditch', focusing on scrips and skills as core practices, to a radical 'constructivist ditch', focusing on freedom and creativity. It seems important to engage student teachers, practicum teachers and teacher educators to reflect on both the potential and limitations of disciplined improvisation, thus developing their knowledge base, their responsibility and accountability and their autonomy.

(11)Abstract The basic impoverishment of deafness is not lack of hearing but lack of language. To illustrate this, we have only to compare a 4-year-old hearing child, with a working vocabulary of between 2,000 and 3,000 words, to a child of the same age, profoundly deaf since infancy, who may have only a few words at his command. Even more important than vocabulary level, however, is the child's ability to use his language for expressing ideas, needs, and feelings. By the age of 4 years, the hearing child in all cultures has already grasped the rules of grammar syntax that enable him or her to combine words in meaningful ways.

2.03) Observations:

Summary and Conclusions

The findings confirm the initial research hypotheses regarding the superior intellectual and social functioning of deaf children with deaf parents, compared to deaf children with hearing parents. Data from Stanford Achievement Tests (reading, arithmetic, and overall grade level), as well as teacher–counselor ratings for intellectual functioning, disclosed significant differences between the sets of matched pairs in the predicted direction. In the area of social functioning, differences favoring children with deaf parents were particularly impressive in areas of behavior that have often been cited as "characteristic" of deaf individuals. These include traits such as maturity, responsibility, independence, sociability, and appropriate sex role behavior.

The results of ratings and speech reading test, measuring communicative functioning, were less clear. No differences were found among children with deaf parents, and those with hearing parents received significantly higher ratings for facility with written language, receptive and expressive finger spelling, and use of the language of signs. On the other hand, various measures of manual communication were positively related to facility in speech reading, as measured by the Craig Inventory. Early oral training seems to be related to later communicative functioning and is less likely to have been experienced by children with deaf parents.

None of the evidence from the research reported above would seem to justify the strong injunctions placed by professional educators on the use of manual communication by parents of young deaf children. Children in this study who had been exposed to early manual communication performed at a higher level by almost every measure employed. This conclusion is not meant to discourage early oral training for deaf children. On the contrary, some evidence was reported to the effect that children who are most likely to be judged as having good communicative skills are those who were exposed to both oral and manual training at an early age.

2.04) Characteristics of the study

The review makes it clear that the programmes for the language development of the hearing impaired were tested. The researcher conducted an experiment to study the following characteristics:

The researcher developed a questionnaire to investigate difficulties in language development faced by the hearing impaired students, their teachers and parents.

The researcher investigates the reasons why do these difficulties occur.

The researcher developed a questionnaire to examine the present ways and methods of language teaching applied by teachers from special school and parents of hearing impaired students with a view to overcoming the difficulties in language development. The researcher executed improvisation technique to test its effectiveness in language development.

The suggestions for the present ways and methods applied by teachers and parents to overcome these difficulties were cross checked.

The important processes for language development of hearing impaired were observed.

The programme was developed and tried out experimentally to test its effectiveness.

The design selected to test the effectiveness of the programme was pretest posttest control group design.

Both the groups were tested by state government's language test. The review of related literature thus helped the researcher to understand the dimensions of language development and the process of developing improvisation technique thereby giving directions to his study.

CHAPTER 2.REFERENCES

1) Dramatization as a Method of Developing Spoken English Skill, International Journal of Language & Linguistics Vol. 1, No. 1; June 2014

2) Research in Drama Education: The Journal of Applied Theatre and Performance, Issue 2, Volume 6, 2001

3) censusindia.gov.in/census_and_you/disabled_population.aspx 2011

4) https://www.ncbi.nlm.nih.gov/pmc/articles/PMC3384464/.Published online 2012 Apr 2

5) http://www.sorich.in/2017/11/overview-of-deaf-literacy-in-india.html

6) https://www.researchgate.net/publication/6976161_Parental_Resources_Parental_Stress_and_Socioemotional_Development_of_Deaf_and_Hard_of_Hearing_Children

7) https://academic.oup.com/jdsde/article/11/4/493/409057,*The Journal of Deaf Studies and Deaf Education*, Volume 11, Issue 4, Fall 2006,

8) https://www.researchgate.net/publication/311215976_Avoiding_Linguistic_Neglect_of_Deaf_Children, December 2016 Social Service Review 90(4):589-619

9) https://pediatrics.aappublications.org/content/136/1/170

10) Pediatrics July 2015, 136 (1) 170-176; DOI: https://doi.org/10.1542/peds.2014-1632

11) Published by Linguistic Society of America DOI: 10.1353/lan.2014.0036

INDEX
CHAPER 3: Methodology

3.00) Paradigm   88

3.01) Introduction   88

3.02) Choice of methods   88

3.03) Population and Sample   89

3.04) Selection of the tool   89

3.05) Timeline of collection of the Data   89

3.06) Description of implementation of the programme   90

3.07) Method of Analysis of the data   92

3.08) Design and Implementation of the Experimental study   92

REFERENCES   102

3.00) Paradigm:

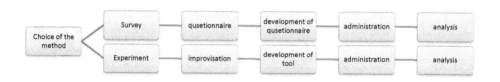

3.01) Introduction:

This chapter describes the process of selection of research methods, selection of tools for data collection, development of the questionnaire, its finalisation process and classification of data and method of data collection.

It is an applied research as its purpose is improving a process. Researcher selected "Pretest posttest control and experimental group design", as the main objective of the experimentation was to test the effectiveness of the training programme. Survey and experiment both were conducted; hence it is mixed method design.

3.02) Choice of methods:

As mentioned in Chapter 1, according to the objectives of the study the researcher wanted

(1) to investigate difficulties in language development faced by the hearing impaired students, their teachers and parents and

(2) to examine the present ways and methods of language teaching applied by teachers from special school and parents of hearing impaired students with a view to overcoming the difficulties in language development.

To fulfil these purposes survey method was selected.

(3) To develop The Improvisation program for hearing impaired students researcher referred booklet (No.15) developed by YCMOU, this depicts about construction of research tool stepwise. This was very helpful as it gave clarity to the researcher about entire process of designing, executing and evaluating research tool.

(4) for testing the effectiveness of improvisation programme in language development pretest-posttest design study was used in which students were observed before and after giving base line test. This study design looks at one group of individuals who receive the intervention through programme, which is called the treatment/experimental group. The pretest-posttest design allows making inferences on the effect of intervention by looking at the difference in the pre-test and post-test results.

3.03) Population and Sample

Population of the study was hearing impaired students from special primary school.

In Pune city area and its suburb, there are 12 special primary schools for 970 deaf students and 108 working teachers. There are 3 residential schools with 150 students, 6 nonresidential schools with 535 students and 3 schools having 285 resident and nonresident students.

Researcher approached these schools for the survey through questionnaire of teachers and parents. Schools governed by Suhrud Mandal, Pune granted the permission to conduct the survey in three schools and to execute the experiment in one school.

For execution of experimental method total 40 students participated from two residential schools. Total 20 parents and 21 teachers participated in the survey.

Taking into consideration the spread of population of students with moderate hearing loss and moderately severe loss, the random selection of the sample for control and experiment will be difficult. So equivalent groups of students were selected and distributed for control and experimental treatment.

For experimental method, experimental group and control group from two different residential schools were selected. These groups were selected by researcher as the required sample was from equal socio, economical and educational background. In experimental group 21 students and in control group 19 students were selected.

3.04) Selection of the tool:

To investigate difficulties in language development faced by the hearing impaired students, their teachers and parents and to examine the present ways and methods of language teaching applied by teachers and parents, the survey was conducted .The researcher use the questionnaire for the teachers and parents. (Appendix A,B). Interviews were also conducted to fulfill the purpose. (Appendix G)

There is no separate test to evaluate writing, vocabulary and comprehension of hearing impaired. Hence the researcher decided to use baseline test made by Government of Maharashtra (Maharashtra Pradhikaran Parishad, 2017) for the experimental method for pretesting and posttesting.(in appendix F).It could be useful for comparing writing, vocabulary and comprehension with normal children in future.

3.05) The Timeline of collection of the data:

01/11/2016 to 31/12/2016 Teacher's questionnaires and interviews

01/11/2016 to 31/12/2016 Parent's questionnaires and interviews

20/09/2017 pre test   Control Group

18/09/2017 pre test Experimental Group

08/10/2017 post test Control Group

07/10/2017 post test Experimental Group

18/09/2017 to 06/10/2017 Programme conducted in Experimental Group

3.06) Description of the programme:

Improvisation as a Teaching Technique for students to

 1) construct trust,

2) support teamwork and better brainstorming,

 3) improve communication and presentation skills,

4) develop creative problem solving,

5) react alertly and decisively to unexpected challenges,

6) be quick on their feet and recognize opportunities as they get up,

 7) expand their comfort level with change and inclination to take risks, and

 8) make their mind to change and encourage a supportive, improvisational philosophy. The students need to learn how to adapt, adjust, listen, observe, agree, support, trust, and think fast.The inclusion of improvisation as a teaching strategy provides an excellent opportunity to teach students these necessary skills, as they increase in their abilities to achieve academic and professional success[1].

Principles of Improvisation:

There are seven principles of improvisation:

1. Trust: In order for a group to be successful and creative, the participants of the group, must to be able to trust one another.

2. Acceptance: Participants must be willing to accept a new idea in order to explore its possibilities. Every participant must accept the offer, build on it, contribute, and discover new ideas. It is this process that harnesses the power of collaboration. 3. Attentive listening: Participants must be responsive of the partners with whom they are co-creating. This leads to increase their understanding of each other and to be able to communicate effectively.

4. Spontaneity: Spontaneity allows participants to initiate words and actions, building trust with the other players. Participants must defer any significant judgment or spirit about what others say.

5. Storytelling: Participants develop the ability to create a collaborative description that connects their dialogue through a story. This process results in memorable content.

6. Nonverbal communication: Participants use facial expressions and body language to help communicate thoughts, nature, and trustworthiness.

7. Warm-ups:Warm-ups provide to develop trust and safe environments, where the participants can feel free. Warm-up activities core on transitioning individuals into an improvisational mode to allow them to improvise verbally and physically.

3.07) Method of analysis of the data

The researcher wanted to investigate difficulties in language development faced by the hearing impaired students, their teachers and parents and, to examine the present ways and methods of language teaching, hence questionnaire were analysed.

To test the effect of the experiment in the present study, statistical methods were adopted to analyze the data along with the graphical representation was also produced for superior interpretation of data.

The 't' statistics was used to determine if there was any significant difference in the pre test and post test scores of base line test in Experimental School & Control School comparing:

1: Writing+Vocabulary scores

2: Comprehension scores

3: Total scores

3.08) Design and Implementation of the Experimental study

1 Introduction

2 Brief description of theoretical base of 'Improvisation Program'

3 Description of the Steps followed for the development of 'Improvisation Program'

Step 1	Role of the training program in the present research
Step 2	Specific objectives of the training program
Step 3	Nature and planning of the training program
Step 4	Construction of the training program
Step 5	Actual training program and its description ('Improvisation Program')
Step 6	Pilot testing of the training program
Step 7	Validity and reliability of the training program
Step 8	Changes in the training program according to the feedback during the pilot study
Step 9	Pretesting and final training program
Step 10	Actual implementation of the training program
Step 11	Relation between objectives and outcomes
Step 12	Conclusions and suggestions

1 Introduction

In Chapter one, Researcher discussed about the research problem. In Chapter two, Researcher shared about different literature reviewed. In Chapter three, methodology of the present research was discussed. In this chapter researcher is elaborating about the experiment 'Improvisation Training Program' conducted. This chapter contains design and planning of the experimental study. This chapter also contains session wise report of intervention conducted with experimental group. This will give lot of clarity about the experiment conducted with the experimental group. As researcher wanted to understand effect of dependent variable that is 'Improvisation Training Program' on dependent variable that is 'language development' of hearing impaired, this training program was designed. While conducting survey, Researcher realized that there is awareness in teachers and parents of to help their students/ children to develop their language. Researcher decided to conduct Improvisation Training Program only with students because of time constraints.

2 Brief description of theoretical base of 'Improvisation Training Program':

Improvisation as a Teaching Technique for students to

1) construct trust,

2) support teamwork and better brainstorming,

3) improve communication and presentation skills,

4) develop creative problem solving,

5) react alertly and decisively to unexpected challenges,

6) be quick on their feet and recognize opportunities as they get up,

7) expand their comfort level with change and inclination to take risks, and

8) make their mind to change and encourage a supportive, improvisational philosophy. The students need to learn how to adapt, adjust, listen, observe, agree, support, trust, and think fast.The inclusion of improvisation as a teaching technique provides an excellent opportunity to teach students these necessary skills, as they increase in their abilities to achieve academic and professional success.

3 Description of steps followed for the development of Training

A series of fifteen booklets is developed by 'Yashwantrao Chavan Maharashtra Open University (YCMOU) for research purpose. Researcher referred booklet (No.15) which depicts about construction of research tool stepwise. This was very helpful as it gave clarity to the researcher about entire process of designing, executing and evaluating research tool. Steps of the construction of improvisation programme are as follows.

Step 1-Role of the training programme in the present research.

Research technique in this research is 'Improvisation Training Program'. This training program is used as an intervention for Experimental group. It helps the participants to develop their language through mental, verbal and physical activities.

Step 2- Specific Objectives of the training programme.

Overall objective of this training program was to develop the expressions through sign language of hearing impaired. To elaborate this step, researcher has mentioned session wise objectives of the Training Program.

Session wise Objectives of the Training Program

Following are the objectives of each session for the students to develop the expressions through sign language

There are total 17 sessions planned in the experimental study.

1) To interact each other and to form a homogeneous group

2) To create awareness of own body, ready for knowing body language

3) To react in proper manner with other members in the group

4) To build self confidence and believe in others

5) To share our thoughts with actions and signs

6) To know the roles of professionals like a painter, a sculptor, a policeman

7) To express the moment with actions without using words

8) To suggest an incident with body language

9) To communicate with others through dialogue

10) To communicate with others through dialogues and property

11) To communicate with others through dialogues, property and music

12) To express abstract concepts through actions like famine, freedom, loyalty

13) To trust one another, to accept and discover new ideas.

14) To allow initiating words and actions, building trust with the other

15) To provide an opportunity to develop trust and safe environments

16) To use facial expressions and body language to help communicate

17) To create a collaborative narrative that connects dialogue through story

Step 3-Nature and Planning of the training programme

Researcher wanted to develop the language of the hearing impaired, so researcher developed this training program. This training program consists of series of techniques such as attention, perception, memory, significance of experiences, time experience, emotional feeling and expression, self-control, body image, and sense of personal identity[1].

Duration of the complete training program was for 17 days. Each session was conducted for 90 minutes. School allotted time to conduct training was 9.30 am to 11.00 am in the morning. Researcher himself conducted this training program. Researcher practices improvisation in academics and dramatics since last forty years, so he himself instructed and helped participants to learn and practice improvisation. School provided the hall and other necessary equipments to conduct this training program.

Step 4- Construction of the training programme

Initially, while designing and constructing Training Program, researcher pursued following process: The researcher is involved in training of improvisation from last forty years. Hence referring previous case studies, working with different school and college groups, helped researcher to short list activities of training program. The researcher referred from drama and improvisation books, programme manual, going through various training programs from internet. Discussion- As the training programme was in process discussion with experts, from the field of Education, improvisation Training Educators. Researcher had listed down activities to be conducted before, during and for practicing technique.

Step 5- Description of the training programme

Outline of Training Program Session

1 Pretesting of the base line test (n=21)

2 Introduction of the research topic

3 Post testing was conducted using base line test (n=21)

Step 6- Pilot testing and Pilot study of the training programme

Before conducting actual experimental study, pilot study was conducted with the group of fifteen (15) participants. Ten (10) sessions were conducted with the sample group to evaluate feasibility, duration, cost, adverse events, and improve upon the study design prior to performance of a full-scale research project[2]. According to the feedback received by the participants of pilot study and experts, further changes were made in the actual experimental study.

Step 7- Validity and reliability of the training programme

Training program was discussed with the experts. Every activity was implemented and the difficulties while implementation were discussed with the pilot group. It was ensured that this training program will be positively affect to develop the expressions through sign language of hearing impaired.

Step 8-Necessasary changes

Necessary changes were made in the improvisation program according to the feedback from participants during the pilot study. According to the feedback received by the experts, researcher made changes. More number of sessions was planned for learning training skills.

Step 9- Pre testing and final training Program

With the help of review of related literature and feedback received from pilot study; final version of design of training program was prepared.

Step 10- Actual Implementation of the training Program

Orientation to the Participants:

Researcher obtained permission from the school Principal to conduct experiment that is 'Training Program'. The researcher explained the purpose of the study to the students and their role in the study. Orientation session was conducted for one clock hour. Some doubts were asked, which were answered by the end of the orientation session.

Session-wise execution and Report of the 'Improvisation Training Program'

Session No – 1:

The objective of this session was pre testing of baseline test.

Twenty one students participated in the pre testing session. This test measures writing, vocabulary, comprehension skills of the language.

Students were asked to write their answers on the answer sheets. The test was made for all primary students in the state of Maharashtra. Though the language of the test was simple; the instructions for writing the answers were given with the help of special teachers. Pre-testing continued for 35 to 40 minutes.

Session No -2:

In this session researcher discussed research topic with the experimental group. Researcher conducted activities about the various concepts regarding language. Students enthusiastically participated in these activities. Then the discussion made students to interact each other and to form a homogeneous group. Later, interaction took place with help of some of these questions: e.g. how we think? How we speak? How we hear? How we learn? This was followed by exercises for 30 minutes.

Session No-3:

This session started with a physical activity. Researcher gave some instructions regarding awareness of our own body, ready for knowing body language of the participants.

Ice braking game like wolf-goat was conducted to interact each other. The participants were divided into two groups. One group was named WOLF and another GOAT. As the researcher calls WOLF, every member from group WOLF tried to catch the member of the group GOAT. All the members from the group GOAT ran away and touched the side wall of the hall. Same procedure is repeated for the GOAT group. After 10 minutes the numbers of more members who can catch the members of another group were declared the winners.

Another activity named mirror image was conducted. In this activity, one member stands in front of all others seated in a hall. Another member comes face to face with first member. First member make an action, the other member imitates the same action like reflection in a mirror. This was conducted for 60 minutes.

Session No-4:

Researcher started training sessions to react in proper manner with other members in the group. Physical movements of own body parts leads to create awareness of own body, ready for knowing body language. All members sit in a circle with the researcher. The first member at the researcher's right mimes and describes his action, and the next member to him repeats that action and then adds a new action of his own. The third one repeats the actions of the first two and then adds one of his own. Each member in the circle must first repeat the actions already shown and then add a new mime. Should he forget an action, give it in the wrong sequence, or identify incorrectly, he is out of the game. The winning member is the last one left in the group. This was conducted for 60 minutes.

Session No- 5:

In this session the researcher conducted the activity to build self confidence and to believe in others. Exercise like Mirror image helped in action and reaction to react in proper manner with other members in the group. There were two players. 'B' is the follower (mirror) and 'A' starts all the action. 'B' reflects all A's movements and facial expressions. Simple activities for 'B' to initiate were combing hair, washing hands, getting dressed, brushing teeth – etc. This exercise promotes inventiveness, clowning, and timing – the children should be encouraged to be as specific as they can with each movement. When "B" is finished, it is "A's" turn. This was practiced for 60 minutes.

Session No- 6:

The exercise to share our thoughts with actions and signs was conducted in this session. Believe in others exercise build self confidence as well as believe in others. The participants formed a circle. One participant will stand in the middle of the circle, closing eyes. After a predetermined signal, the participant in the centre will stiffen his/her body and fall forward, backward or wherever toward the participants standing in closed circle. It's their job to gently catch the blind participant and keep from hitting the ground. As participants became more comfortable with one another, the distance between them can be increased. This was practiced for 60 minutes.

Session No-7:

This session was conducted to know the roles of professionals like a painter, a sculptor, and a policeman.Participants were divided into groups. One group presented their activity, while other were observing. The participant from one group started miming the actions of his/her allocated professional. Other group members joined with related and supportive actions with the first. These theatrical games and team building exercises were executed to share thoughts with actions and signs.This was enjoyed for 60 minutes.

Session No-8:

To represent the object/article with actions without using words. Participants were divided into small groups of between four and six. The idea of the exercise was to get the groups to create the object in ten seconds. Objects can be categorized into: mechanical tools, kitchen objects, garden equipments, school furniture, bathroom accessories etc. Some of the groups were prepared to do this with animals. It was also a great warm up team game. This was conducted for 60 minutes.

Session No-9:

To suggest an incident with body language. Everyone moved around the hall, jumping, skipping, walking anything that was energetic, along with music, then shout and show the placard of the word 'freeze'. Whatever position they were in they must justify by making that position work and taking it into a scene. (e.g. a person stopped with his/her right arm stretched up and left hand lowered, it could be an action of a badminton player.) This game was done with just the facial expression; on 'freeze' they used the expression to create a character. This was conducted for 60 minutes.

Session No-10:

To communicate with others through dialogue: Participants were divided into groups; the subject selected in the script was related with the emotions and familiar words with each group. The script had less importance in drapery, makeup, etc. The script demanded more on imagination and spontaneous acting style. The dialogues were practiced with pauses, pitch variations, loudness of volume with emotions accordingly. Every student was corrected in speech using his/her individual hearing aid. This was practiced for 60 minutes.

Session No-11:

to communicate with others through dialogues and property. Participants were divided into groups; the subject selected was related with the experiences and familiar words with each group. The presentation using different types of property included actions simultaneously. It was an exercise from experimental theatre; it gave opportunity to creativity in students through live and verbal presentation. Every student was corrected in speech using his/her individual hearing aid; the dialogues were practiced in proper manner according to each character played.This was practiced for 60 minutes.

Session No-12:

to communicate with others through dialogues, property and live music. The basic technique of drama was introduced to the team including how to stand with the co-actor and face the audience. Inhaling and exhaling of breathing was exercised during speech, the movements on the stage were worked out along with facial expressions, eye contacts, use of properties and musical instruments.This was practiced for 60 minutes.

Session No-13:

to express abstract concepts through actions like famine, freedom, loyalty. Entire team comes on stage. A scene based on an abstract concept was given to them and within stipulated time all have to form a statue depicting the given scene. The scene was shot on mobile camera and shown to entire group. The discussion was conducted on right and wrong parts of the scene. Taking valuable suggestions the proper scene was depicted again with the help of same participants. This was practiced for 60 minutes.

Session No-14:

to trust one another and accept and discover new ideas. Participants were divided into pairs. Two students act out a scene with standing behind each other. One student stands behind the other, sticking his arms through the arms of the front student, becoming his hands. The student stands in front gave facial or verbal expressions and the student at the back made the hand gestures relatively. This was followed by practice for 60 minutes.

Session No-15:

to allow initiating words and actions, building trust with the other. All participants carried out a series of verbal commands e.g. walk slowly, fly, run etc. This was followed by practice for 60 minutes.

Session No-16:

to provide an opportunity to develop trust and safe environments .Each participant was encouraged to volunteer for all the above activities. Everyone began to realise that what they say and do is important to other. The importance of these activities lies in the process and not in the product. This was followed by practice for 60 minutes.

Session No-17:

to use facial expressions and body language to help communicate. Each participant learned to use all parts of the body to express the different actions. Every single action was clearly and precisely presented so that it was easily identified. This was followed by practice for 60 minutes

Session No-18:

to create a collaborative narrative that connects dialogue through story. Participants seat in a circle. One participant told a sentence. Then anti clockwise each one adds his/her sentence. This was followed until one story is evolved through .This can be repeated several times for different topics.

Session No-19:

The objective of this session was post testing of baseline test.

Twenty one students participated in the post testing session. This test measures writing, vocabulary, comprehension skills of the language.

Table No: 3.1 shows the session wise summary of activities conducted by the researcher:

Day	Date	Technique	Activity	Purpose
Session 1	18/09/2017	Pre test	Writing test	To measure the skills like writing, vocabulary and comprehension
Session 2	18/09/2017	Ice braking	Games like wolf-goat, mirror image	To interact each other and to form a homogeneous group
Session 3	19/09/2017	Physical	Movements of own body parts	To create awareness of own body, ready for knowing body language
Session 4	20/09/2017	Mirror image	Action and reaction	To react in proper manner with other members in the group
Session 5	21/09/2017	Believe in others	Building confidence	To build self confidence and believe in others
Session 6	22/09/2017	Theatrical games	Team building exercises	To share our thoughts with actions and signs
Session 7	23/09/2017	Drawings	Self expressions	To know the roles of professionals

		Improvisation	Enact	like a painter, a sculptor, a policeman
Session 8	25/09/2017	Improvisation	Incidents using mime	To express the moment with actions without using words
Session 9	26/09/2017	Improvisation	Composition-Structured frame	To suggest an incident with body language
Session 10	27/09/2017	Improvisation	Enact concrete incident	To communicate with others through dialogue
Session 11	28/09/2017	Improvisation	Enact concrete incident	To communicate with others through dialogues and property
Session 12	29/09/2017	Improvisation	Enact concrete incident	To communicate with others through dialogues, property and music
Session 13	30/09/2017	Theatrical games	Enact abstract images	To express abstract concepts through actions like famine, freedom, loyalty
Session 14	02/10/2017	Improvisation	Trust. Acceptance	To trust one another. To accept and discover new ideas.
Session 15	03/10/2017	Improvisation	Spontaneity	To allow to initiate words and actions, building trust with the other
Session 16	04/10/2017	Improvisation Role playing	Warm-ups	To provide an opportunity to develop trust and safe environments
Session 17	05/10/2017	Improvisation Role playing	Nonverbal communication	To use facial expressions and body language to help communicate
Session 18	06/10/2017	Improvisation	Storytelling	To create a collaborative narrative that connects dialogue through story
Session 19	07/10/2017	Post test	Writing test	To measure the skills like writing, vocabulary and comprehension

Step 11- Relation between objectives and outcome: The analysis of relation between objectives and outcome is mentioned in detail in Chapter 5-Data Analysis and Data Interpretation.

Step 12- Conclusions and Suggestions

Conclusions and Suggestions regarding this training programme are mentioned in Chapter 5.

Research study at a glance:

No.	Objective	Research method	Population/ Sample size	Data collection tool	Data analysis tool
1	To investigate difficulties in language development faced by the hearing impaired students, their teachers and parents	Survey	20 parents 21 teachers	Questionnaires for teachers and parents, Interviews by teachers and parents,	Frequency table
2	To examine the present ways and methods of language teaching applied by teachers from special school and parents of hearing impaired students with a view to overcoming the difficulties in language development.	Survey	20 parents 21 teachers	Questionnaires for teacher educators and parents, Interviews by teacher educators and parents,	Frequency table
3	To develop the improvisation programme for hearing impaired students	-	-	-	-
4	To test the effectiveness of improvisation technique in language development	Experiment	Control group= 19 Experimental Group= 21	Baseline test made by Government of Maharashtra (Maharashtra Pradhikaran Parishad, 2017)	't' statistics for hypothesis Graphs

INDEX
CHAPTER 4: Analysis and Interpretation

4.00) Paradigm 104

4.01) Introduction 104

4.02) Analysis of data obtained by the Survey: 104

A) Analysis of data obtained from teacher's questionnaires 104

B) Analysis of data obtained from parent's questionnaires 120

4.03) Analysis of data obtained by the Experiment: 153

A) Analysis of data obtained by Experimental group 154

B) Analysis of data obtained by Control Group 157

C) Analysis of data for comparison of Experimental and Control 161
Groups

4.04) Testing the Hypothesis: 164

A) Testing of the Hypothesis 1 165

B) Testing of the Hypothesis 2 166

C) Testing of the Hypothesis 3 167

4.00) Paradigm:

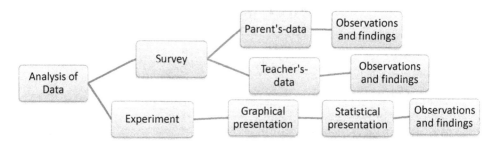

4.01) Introduction:

In Chapter one researcher discussed about the research problem. In Chapter two, researcher shared about different literature reviewed. In Chapter three, methodology of the present research was discussed.

In this chapter researcher is elaborating about the survey and the experiment 'Improvisation' conducted. The chapter contains design and planning of the survey and the experimental study.

4.02) Analysis of data obtained by Survey :

This section describes the analysis of data obtained by Survey to relate the major research questions of the survey. The researcher wanted 1) to investigate difficulties in language development faced by the hearing impaired students, their teachers and parents, 2) to examine the present ways and methods of language teaching.

Hence 20 parents and 21 teachers of moderate and severe hearing impaired children from the special school were selected for questionnaire and interviews. The students of those parents and teachers were learning from pre-primary to 7th Std. in special schools of Pune city and suburb area. Information about severity of deafness, efforts taken by parents, teachers through formal and informal education was collected by the data.While conducting survey; Researcher realized that there is awareness of extra efforts taken for language development by teachers and parents of the deaf children.

A) Analysis of data obtained from Teacher's Questionnaire:

Table 4.001

Gender wise description of the teachers:

Gender	No.
Female:	13
Male:	08
Total	21

Total teachers are 21. All are from special schools.13 out of 21 teachers are female and 8are male. This is the representation from most of the special Group, that majority is the female teachers. The reason may be they are more sensitive, aware of needs and difficulties of this age group, have more patience, carries motherly attitude in any situation, sympathetic in nature, talkative, along with the characteristics of good teacher.

Table 4.002

Educationl qualification of the teachers:

Qualification	No.
Up to 12th std	02
Graduate	13
Post graduate:	06
Total	21

13 out of 21 teachers are graduate, 6are post graduate and 2 are literate up to 12th standard. All are qualified and most of them have their knowledge base is wide in their subject.

Table 4.003

Teaching experience of the teachers:

No. Of years	No.
00 to 05 years	02
05 to 10 years	07

10 to 15 years	05
More than 15 yrs	06
No response	01
Total	21

2 teachers have up to 5 years of teaching experience,7 teachers have up to 10years of teaching experience,5 teachers have up to 15 years of teaching experience,6 teachers have more than of 15 years teaching experience,1 gives no response. The percentage of experienced teacher, i. e. more than 10 years, is more. It indicates that more expertise is used in teaching learning process, enriched inputs are given, innovative ways are explored for co-curricular activities, and students get more exposure in different fields, long term interaction with parents this results positively on the academic performance of the students.

Table 4.004

Levels of teaching sections

Level of students	No.
Pre primary	12
Primary	12
Higher primary	07
Secondary	06
No response	01

12 teachers are working for pre primary level, 12 teachers are working for primary level, 7 teachers are working for higher primary level, 6 teachers are working for secondary level, and 1 gives no response. Majority of the teachers have experience of dealing with age appropriate curriculum and understanding the learning level of the student. The teachers are more in numbers, in pre primary and primary levels. It indicates that the number of teachers decreases at upper levels, because of less numbers of students in higher primary and secondary levels.

Table 4.005

Qualification in Special education:

Qualification	No.
Diploma	05
Graduate	16
Post graduate	01
Other	01

5 teachers are diploma holder, 16 got degree in special education, 1 is post graduate and 1 didn't respond. All 21 teachers got certified education in their specialized field, i.e. hearing impairment. All are well qualified in their respective field. They are aware of the special needs of the students; trained in language acquisition, language learning, along with their all round development with appropriate age group. Teachers have more subject expertise, well informed and practiced in new technology, experienced in content and methodology.

Table 4.006

Language teaching equipment:

Name of the equipment	No.
Individual hearing aid	19
Speech trainer	07
Group hearing aid	03
Other(FM)	06

19 teachers uses individual hearing aid, 7 uses speech trainer, 3 uses group hearing aid, 6 uses frequency modulation. It indicates the awareness of using advanced technology in teaching learning process. High tech equipments are used with appropriate hearing loss. The basic necessities of hearing impaired are fulfilled with these equipments.

Table 4.007

Sources used for language learning other than books:

Name of the source	No.
Internet	03
Pictured books	10
Computer / e-learning	17
Requirements(expt.)	01
Projector	01
News paper	03
Dramatization	04
Charts	11
Models	08
Word chits	11
Actual experiences	03
Google apps	01
Mobile phone	02
No response	02

03teachers uses Internet, 10 uses Pictured books,17 uses Computer / e-learning, 01 uses
Requirements (expt.), 01 uses Projector, 03 uses News paper, 04 uses Dramatization, 11 uses
Charts, 08 uses Models, 11 uses Word chits, 03 gives Actual experiences, 01 uses Google apps,
02 uses Mobile phone, 02gives no response. There is a large range of the sources used by the
teachers for language learning other than books.The teachers are user friendly with new
technology and experienced in advance technology. Variation in sources builds the base of the
thought in language development of the children.

Table 4.008

Creation of educational aids

Created by teachers	No.
Yes	19
No	01
No response	01

19 teachers create their own educational aids, 1 didn't create, 1 didn't respond. Most of the teachers understand the audiogram of their students. Hence they are aware of their residual hearing; accordingly they can prepare need based learning material. This shows the creativity of the teacher.

Table 4.009

Usefulness when used by others

Useful	No.
Yes	20
Used by himself	01

20 teachers experiences advantage of educational material when used by others,1 used by himself. Most of the teachers experiences that it is useful for other students also, when used by their colleagues; it indicates the validity and reliability of the material.

Table 4.010

Sharing of educational material

Sharing with other teachers	No.
Yes	19
No	02

19 teachers shared the educational aid with others, 2 doesn't share. It shows the co-operative nature of the teacher, eagerness to trying on different levels and readiness to experimentation.

Table 4.011

Opinions of other teachers about sharing

Opinions about sharing	No.
No answer/reaction	03
Liked	04
Suggestions for betterment	03
Used whenever as it is saved	02
Good response from students	09
Useful as per hearing loss	01
Facilitates teaching learning	03
Language development occurs	01
Useful for fixation	01
No response	02

03 teachers gives no answer/reaction, 04 liked, 03 gives suggestions for betterment,02 used whenever as it can be saved, 09 have good response from students, 01experiences useful as per hearing loss, 03 facilitates teaching learning, 01language development occurs, 01 finds useful for fixation, 02 gives no response . It shows the usefulness of the material and readiness to alter the material.

Table 4.012

Student's favorite activity for language learning

Name of the activity	No.
About cleanliness	01
Sign language	02
Reading/to search words from newspaper	03
Related to science	01

Short sentences	01
e-learning	02
Activity lesson	01
Picture medium	04
Dramatization	02
Kar pallawi	01
To solve puzzles	02
Learn through play	01
To make words	02
Book reading	01
Information about leaders/festivals	02

01 student likes activity about cleanliness, 02 students likes Sign language, 03 likes Reading/to search words from newspaper,01 likes activity Related to science, 01 likes Short sentences, 02 likes activity e-learning, 01 likes Activity lesson, 04 likes Picture medium, 02 likes activity Dramatization, 01 likes Kar pallawi, 02 likes activity To solve puzzles, 01 likes Learn through play, 02 likes activity To make words, 01 likes Book reading, 02 likes activity information about leaders/festivals. This shows the variation in activities for language development.Activities like picture medium, dramatization, learn through play, make words incline to raise the vocabulary.

Table 4.013

Reason to like the activity

Reason to like the activity	No.
New knowledge is generated	03
Helps in language growth	03

Remember the incidence orderly	01
Active participation	05
Helps in writing	02
Opportunity for different role-play	04
Appraisal	01
Good for practice	02
Versatile/variety	02
Language learning by visuals	01
No response	01

03 students likes activity because New knowledge is generated, 03 students likes activity because it Helps in language growth, 01 students likes activity because it Remember the incidence orderly, 05 students likes activity because of Active participation, 02 students likes activity because it Helps in writing, 04 students likes activity because opportunity for different role-play, 01 students likes for Appraisal, 02 students likes activity because it is Good for practice, 02 students likes activity because of variety, 01 students likes activity because Language learning by visuals, 01 gives no response. Teacher knows how to perform activity and how to conduct it. But if there is knowledge of why it is conducted, then it is fruitful.

Table 4.014

Teacher's belief about student's language

Learning by teaching	No.
Yes	12
No	07
No response	02

12 Teachers believes that students learn language by teaching, 07 teachers says no,They learn on their own and 02 teachers gives no response. Actually children learn language on their own.Language can be acquired through experiences and observations.

Table 4.015

Teacher's observations about student's language

Mode of language learning	No.
Owned their collection of words	01
Read and write short sentences	03
Learn through environment	04
Don't know before Grouping	04
Can't hear words due to hearing loss	04
Expresses feelings through signs, we teach language	02
No response	02

01 teacher observed that Owned their collection of words, 03 teachers observed that students Read and write short sentences, 04 teachers observed that students Read Learn through environment, 04 teachers observed that students Read Don't know before Grouping, 04 teachers observed that students Read Can't hear words due to hearing loss, 02 teachers observed that students Read Expresses feelings through signs, we teach language, 02 teachers gives no response. This happens because, one who can't hear, can't speak. There may be a misconception that, if there is no speech, there is no language.

Table 4.016

Parent's participation in language development of their children

Participates in language development	No.
Yes	12

No	07
Rarely	01

12 parents try for language development, 07 don't, and 01 rarely tries. The child spent more time with the parents, therefore there is a wide communication and chance of greater opportunities for language development in the company of parents.

Table 4.017

Parent's efforts in language development of their children

Efforts by parents	No.
Less	18
More	01
No response	02

18 teachers say fewer efforts are taken by parents, 01 says more efforts are taken by parents, 02 gives no response. Less no. of parents are involved in language development of their children. How much time can spare parents with their children will possibly develop the language.

Table 4.018

Type of efforts observed by parents for language development

Observed efforts by parents	No.
Learn language of hearing impaired	04
Write word chits on articles at home	07
Learn sign language	03
Continuous conversation with child	08
Revision at home	05
Spend more time for favorite subject	01
Teach the maintenance the hearing aid	04

Need based efforts	03
Develop habit of hearing different voices	02
Inform different subjects	01
Learn through experiences	02
Early entrance in the Group	01
Use of pictured notebook/book	01
No response	01

04 teachers observed that parents Learn language of hearing impaired, 07 teachers observed that parents Write word chits on articles at home, 03 teachers observed that parents Learn sign language, 08 teachers observed that parents continuously conversee with child, 05 teachers observed that parents take Revision at home, 01 teacher observed that parents Spend more time for favorite subject, 04 teachers observed that parents Teach the maintenance the hearing aid, 03 teachers observed that parents take Need based efforts, 02 teachers observed that parents Develop habit of hearing different voices, 01 teacher observed that parents Inform different subjects, 02 teachers observed that parents Learn through experiences, 01 teacher observed that parents have Early entrance in the Group, 01 teacher observed that parents uses pictured notebook/book, 01 gives no response. It reflects the concepts about the language development of the parents; their awareness about the activities for the same without the books. Language development is beyond the school syllabi and the books.

Table 4.019

Awareness of parents for language development in other countries

Parents are aware	No.
Yes	11
No	04
No response	03

11 teachers observed awareness of parents about other practices, 04 teachers didn't, 03 give no response. Parents are aware of different ways, techniques or technology other than in our country.

Table 4.020

Formats of awareness of parents

Formats of awareness	No.
Sign language	13
Oral	11
Total communication	08
Oral aural	05
Kar pallawi	01
Audio visual	06
e-learning	02
Qued speech	02
No response	04

13 parents uses Sign language,11 parents uses Oral exercise,08 parents uses Total communication,05 parents uses Oral aural method,01 parent uses Kar pallawi,06 parents uses Audio visual,02 parents uses E-learning,02 parents uses Qued speech.04 gives no response.

The alternatives can be used by parents. Different possible ways can guide the child to develop the language.

Table 4.021

Conduction of workshops

Conduction of workshops	No.
Yes	19

No	01
No response	01

19 Teachers says Workshops are conducted for parents by Schools, 01 says No, and 01 gives no response. Workshops are meant to enrich the parents in new knowledge and technology.

Table 4.022

Workshops benefits the parents

Benefit to parents	No.
Yes	16
No	03
Not sure	01
No response	02

16 parents agree benefit of workshops, 03 say No, 01 is Not sure, 02 gives no response. Workshops benefit the parents. There are some guided programmes for the development of the children.

Table 4.023

Hobbies of the teachers

Hobbies	No.
Reading	14
Singing	01
Roaming	01
Learn new things	03
Articles/ picture collection	06
Dance	02

Computer	01
Games	05
Preparation of educational aids	01
Write poems	01
Exercise/work out	01
Travel	03
Swimming	01
Gardening	01
Watch T.V.	02
No response	01

14 teachers have hobby of Reading, 01 teacher have hobby of Singing, 01 teacher have hobby of Roaming, 03 teachers have hobby of learning new things, 06 teachers have hobby of collecting Articles/ picture,02 teachers have hobby of dancing,01 teachers have hobby of Computer learning,05 teachers have hobby of playing Games,01 teacher have hobby of Preparation of educational aids,01 teacher have hobby of writing poems,01 teacher have hobby of Exercise/work out,03 teachers have hobby of travelling,01 teacher have hobby of Swimming, 01 teachers have hobby of Gardening,02 teachers have hobby to Watch T.V.,01 gives no response.

It can be co- relate with the co-curricular activity. It reflects the interest of the teacher, mainly the type of sharing with the students. Reading, singing, dances, and games like activities are good for mental and physical health. These are also good habits for personality development.

Table 4.024

Hobbies enhances teaching

Ways of enhancement through hobbies	No.
In different projects	02

Provoke different thoughts	03
Preparing note book of different cuttings	04
Preparation of ppt	02
Useful in games	01
Practice in drawing	02
Students learn happily	01
Poems can learn rhythmically	01
Useful in showing pictures in different subjects	03
Create interest in learning new skills	02
Can mention references/context	06
Useful in story telling	02
Cognition of concepts	03
Helps in language growth	02
Dancing helps in exercise and freshness	02
Closeness and kindness with students	01
No response	03

02 help teachers think hobbies In different projects,03 teachers think hobbies Provoke different thoughts,04 teachers think hobbies help Preparing note book of different cuttings,02 teachers think hobbies help in Preparation of ppt,01 teachers think hobbies are Useful in games,02 teachers think hobbies helps in Practice in drawing,01 teachers think hobbies helps in Students happy learning,01 teacher think hobbies helps in teaching Poems learn rhythmically,03 teachers think hobbies are Useful in showing pictures in different subjects,02 teachers think hobbies helps in creating interest in learning new skills,06 teachers think hobbies helps in references/context,02

119

teachers think hobbies helps are Useful in story telling,03 teachers think hobbies helps in Cognition of concepts,02 teachers think hobbies helps in language growth,02 teachers think hobby of Dancing helps in exercise and freshness,01 teacher think hobbies helps in Closeness and kindness with students,03gives no response. The exploration of different ways of enhancement through hobbies was tested by the teachers. Above range of activities shows the creativity and interest of the teacher. The list opens new avenues in language teaching.

B) Analysis of data obtained from Parent's questionnaire

1. Out of 20 wards 11 are male, 09 are female. The number of parents having male students than female students is more.

2. Education of students: 09 students are learning in pre-primary and 11 in primary level.

Table 4.025

Educational Background of family members

| Person   in | Number | Illiterate | Primary | Secondary |
family				
Father	09	-	03	06
Mother	09	03	01	05
Brother	04	02	02	-
Sister	06	-	03	03

Most of the family members are passed from secondary school, 09 are passed from primary school and 05 are illiterate.

Table 4.026

Economical background

Yearly income of family in Rs.	Number
10,000 to 50,000	03
50,000 to 1,00,000	03

More than 1,00,000	01
No response	13

Yearly income of 03 families is in between Rs.10,000 to Rs.50,000,03 families in between Rs.50,000 to Rs.1,00,000,03,01 family have More than Rs.1,00,000, ,13of them gives no response. The respondents are from very low income group. The status of most of the families has very low socio-economic background.

Table 4.027

Observed span of hearing test

Time span	No.
Before 1st year	03
After 1st year	07
After 2nd year	02
After 3rd year	06
No response	02

03 parents observed hearing test of a child before completing 1st year, 07 parents after 1st year, 02 parents after 2nd year, 06 parents after 3rd year, and 02 parents gives no response. Most of the parents diagnosed the hearing loss before the 3rd year, which is a critical period for language development. This is very valuable period for developing and learning any language.

Table4.028

Get informed about the test

By whom	No.
Self	13
Relatives	01
Group teacher	02

Other (doctor)	02
No response	02

13 parents get informed about the test by themselves, 01by Relatives, 02 parents by Group teacher, 02 parents by other (doctor), and 02parents gives no response. Most of the parents are early aware of the deafness themselves.

Table4.029

By whom it is tested

By whom	No.
Expert	18
School	01
No response	01

18 students are tested by Expert, 01 student is tested by school, 01gives no response. Most of the children are tested by experts. This shows the authenticity in early years.

Table 4.030

Confirmation of Report

Confirmation	No.
Yes	18
No response	02

18parents confirmed the reports, 02gives no response. Report of the diagnosis was confirmed by the experts, the deafness was accepted by parents.

Table 4.031

Person confirms the report

By whom	No.
Expert	20

Expert confirms all 20 reports. Reports of the correct diagnosis of all the children were confirmed by the expert.

Table 4.032

Type of hearing loss

Type	No.
Conductive	10
Sensory-neural	07
No response	03

10 students have Conductive hearing loss, 07 have Sensory-neural hearing loss, 03 gives no response. Parents get the knowledge of type of deafness and its characteristics. Most of the children have conductive hearing loss, where hearing aid may help in limit. Sensory-neural hearing loss is not repairable.

Table 4.033

Ear having hearing loss

Which ear	No.
Left	01
Both	19

01 child have hearing loss in Left ear, 19 have in both the ears. Most of the children have hearing loss in both the ears. Parents confirm the information about deafness.

Table 4.034

Range of hearing loss	Left ear	Right ear
25dB to 40dB	-	-
41dB to 60dB	01	01
More than 61dB	16	15
No response 03		

16 children have hearing loss more than 61dB in both the ears, 03 gives No response. Most of the children have moderate or severe hearing loss. There is residual hearing according to hearing impairment which results into possible language development.

Table 4.035

Necessity of hearing aid

Necessity of aid	No.
Yes	19
No	01

19parents are aware of hearing aid, 01 is not aware. Majority of parents are well-aware   that hearing aid is necessary for their child. They know the benefits of the hearing aid.

Table 4.036

Type of hearing aid

Type of aid	No.
Behind the ear	16
In the ear	04

16 children use behind the ear, 04 children use in the ear type of hearing aids. Behind the ear hearing aid is widely used by the children, suitable device according to diagnosis.

Table 4.037

Regular use of hearing aids

Consistency	No.
Yes	16
No	04

16students constantly uses aid, 04 students didn't use constantly. Hearing aid is used consistently by majority of children, possibly benefits more.

Table 4.038

Use of the hearing aids after diagnosis

Acted immediately	No.
Yes	13
No	07

13 parents acted immediately after diagnosis, 07 didn't act. Most of the children were immediately supported by the hearing aid after diagnosis. Acceptance of impairment and remedial action had been taken immediately by parents.

Table 4.039

Sounds audible without aids

Type of sound	No.
Human	04
By other machines	14
Don't know	01
No sound	01
No response	02

04 children have human sounds audible without aids, 14 have other machine's sounds audible without aids, 01 is unaware, 01cannot hear sound, 02 gives no response. Most of the mechanical sounds are audible than human voice to the children. Not always supportive for language development.

Table 4.040

Awareness about other type of test

Awareness	No.
No	20

No one knows another type of audiometric test. All are unaware of the diagnosis at that age.

Table 4.041

Type of test done

Type of test	No.
No response	20

No one responds to the type of audiometric test. Not aware of new technology, affordable technique.

Table 4.042

Repetition of test

Repetition of test	No.
Yes	07
No	11
No response	02

Test is repeatedly done by 07, Test is not repeatedly done by 11, 02 of them gives no response. Majority of them did not undergo the test. Up to certain age group the test is frequently done.

Table 4.043

Frequency of test

Frequency	No.
1 yearly	06
2 yearly	02
3 yearly	01
No response	11

06 of them are tested 1 yearly, 02 of them are tested 2 yearly, 01 of them is tested 3 yearly, 11 of them gives no response. Very less among them tests the hearing loss frequently. Early intervention may benefit the language development.

Table 4.044

Impact on Hearing loss

126

Impact on loss	No.
decreased	04
increased	03
No change	08
No response	05

04observes decreased in loss, 03observed increased in loss, 08 of them had no change, 05of them gives no response. After testing the hearing loss majority observes no change in hearing.

It shows the observed impact on natural hearing loss.

Table 4.45

Reason behind hearing loss

Reason	No.
Less weight	01
Went to School	02
Can't hear	01
Jaundice	01
No response	13

01 thinks reason behind hearing loss is, less weight,02 thinks reason behind hearing loss is due to mix in school,01,Can't hear,01 thinks reason behind hearing loss is,jaundice,13gives no response. Most of the parents are unaware of the cause of hearing loss. Not knowing the cause effect relationship.

Table 4.046

Responses of the child are recorded

Recording of responses	No.
Yes	11

No	08
No response	01

Responses of the child are recorded by 11parents, 08 parents didn't record, 01gives no response. Most of the parents keep the records of responses given by their child. The change in responses leads to change in practice.

Table 4.047

Mode of recording the responses

Mode of record	No.
In written	01
By graphs	01
Progress card	10
Child's actions	04
School record	05
A/V recording	03
In memory	01
No recordings	01
No response	04

01 child is recorded in written form,01 is recorded by graphs,10 children are recorded through progress card,04 are recorded by child's actions,05 are recorded in school record,03 are recorded by A/V recording,01 keeps in memory,01don't have recordings,04gives no response.

The school record in the form of progress card is supposed to be the main mode of child's record. Language development of a child shows the involvement of parents, teachers, and environment.

Table 4.048

Change in child's speech

change	No.
Yes	16
No	04

16 parents observe change in child's speech, 04 of them didn't. Many parents observed the positive change in speech of the child, while attending the school. They know the level of language of their child.

Table 4.049

Interaction with other parents

Interaction with others	No.
Yes	13
No	06
No response	01

13 parents are connected with other parents. 06 are not min touch with other, 01 gives no response. Many parents have interaction with other parents. Hence they get more information other than their knowledge.

Table 4.050

Reasons of obstacles in the contacts with others

Reason of obstacle	No.
Long distance	01
No obstacle	02
Couldn't sign	01
No response	16

01 feels long distance is the reason for not getting contacts, 02 didn't feel obstacle, 01 couldn't sign, and 16 gives no response. Most of them did not respond about reason of obstacles in contacts with other. No follow-up is observed.

Table 4 .051

Taking care of hearing aid

Caring of aid	No.
Yes	15
No	02
No use of aid	01
No response	02

15 of them take care of hearing aid, 02 didn't, 01 feels no use of aid, 02 gives no response.
Many children can take good care of his/her hearing aid. They know the importance of the device.

Table 4.052

Sufficient training to take care of aid

Training of child	No.
Yes	14
No	03
No response	03

14 children are trained to take care of aid, 03 aren't trained, 03gives no response. Many are trained to take care of hearing aid. Child realises importance of the device. Child is aware of how and why it is to be handled carefully.

Table 4.053

Maintenance of hearing aid

Maintenance of aid	No.
Yes	17
No	01

No response	02

Aid is regularly maintained by 17 children, not maintained by 01,02gives no response. Many of them can maintain the hearing aid regularly. They realises the need and importance of the equipment.

Table 4.054

Financial arrangement for hearing aid

Financial arrangement	No.
Yes	11
No	05
No response	04

11 have financial arrangement for aid, 05 don't have, 04gives no response. Most of them have financial arrangement for maintenance of hearing aid. Knows the importance of necessity requires sufficient funding.

Table 4.055

Financial help for hearing aid

Mode of finance	No.
Yes	05
No	13
No response	02

05of them got financial help for maintenance of aid, 13didn't get financial help, 02gives no response. Most of them do not have economical support for maintenance of hearing aid. They are ready to invest on their own.

Table 4.056

Cleanliness and health of ear

Health care	No.

Yes	19
No	01

19 children care about their ear and health, 01ignores. Everyone is conscious about ear and its cleanliness. Child knows the importance of caring for health.

Table 4.057

Necessity of extra efforts for language development

Necessity of more efforts	No.
Yes	20

All 20 agree that along with hearing loss more efforts taken for language development are necessary. Everyone is aware of extra efforts to be taken for language development and tries to achieve the goals/objectives/landmarks of the language development.

Table 4.058

Spending of sufficient time

Time required	No.
Yes	16
No	04

16 of them have sufficient time for extra efforts, 04 of them cannot spare time. Most of them give sufficient time for language development .Parents know their responsibility and aware in their duties.

4.059

Consumption of time

Time given	No.
1 hr per day	17
No time	01
No response	02

17of them gives, 1 hr per day for language development, 01 don't have time, 02gives no response. Majority of them spends one hour daily for extra efforts to language development. They know the value of the time given for language development.

4.060

Involvement of other family members

Help from other members	No.
Yes	14
No	05
No response	01

14 Of them get help from family members, 05don't get the help, 01gives no response. There is a major involvement of family members in most of the families. The team is working for the development.

Table 4.061

Involved person

Helping person	No.
Mother	15
Father	09
Sister	04
Brother	06
Relative	01
All members	01
No response	03

15 children get help by mother, 09 by father, 04 by sister, 06 by brother, 01 by relative, 01 by all members of family, 03gives no response. In most of the families the mother is the most involved person for language development of a child. Other members and relatives also are interested.

Table 4.062

Another person in the family having hearing loss

History of loss	No.
Yes	01
No	19

Only 1 child has history of hearing loss in his family. In most of the cases there is no history of deafness in the family.

Table 4.063

A person having hearing loss in the family

Person having history	No.
Relative	01
No response	19

01 relative was the person having history of hearing loss, 19 gives no response. Only one family have a case of deafness in their relation. No hereditary or other reasons in rest of the families.

Table 4.064

Opportunity to speak

Opportunity to speak	No.
Yes	15
No	04
No response	01

15 children have opportunity to speak, 04 don't, 01gives no response. Most of the children have opportunity to speak freely.

Table 4.065

Where the child gets the opportunity

Location of opportunity	No.

At home	15
In functions	07
Out of the house	06
No response	04

15 children get opportunity at home, 07 children in functions, 06 children out of the house, 04 gives no response. Most of the children feel free to talk at home. Members at home keep the environment free to learn.

Table 4.066

Child is communicated face to face

Face to face communication	No.
Yes	15
No	05

15 children have face to face communication, 05 don't have. Many children communicate face to face with family members. This is the basic need of every hearing impaired person.

Table 4.067

Communicated through play way

Communication by play	No.
Yes	13
No	07

13 were communication by play, 07 weren't. Play way is the most adopted source for communication. For any type of learning play way is effective method.

Table 4.068

Use of sufficient words for daily routine

Level of vocabulary	No.
Yes	09

No	11

Level of vocabulary of 09 is good, 11 of them have poor level of vocabulary. Most children have poor level of vocabulary. Do not have sufficient vocabulary for daily routine.

Table 4.069

Pace for learning

Own pace of learning	No.
Yes	16
No	04

16 children have their own pace of learning, 04 don't have. Many children take their own pace for learning. Every child has different pace for learning.

Table 4.070

Change of pace observed

Pace is changed	No.
Yes	03
No	14
No response	03

03 are compelled to change their pace, 14 have freedom with their pace, 03 gives no response. Many of them have freedom to keep their own pace though expected pace of learning is not maintained. Many of them do not feel obstacles during their learning.

Table 4.071

Well responded to feelings of child

Responses	No.
Yes	16
No	04

16 of them are treated well in responding to their feelings, 04 are not treated well. In many families children are responded with caring. Language learning need simple and safe atmosphere at home.

Table 4.072

Treated as a normal child

Treatment	No.
Yes	18
No	02

18 are treated as a normal child, 02 are treated as special children. In spite of their deafness most of the children are treated as a normal child. They are not overprotected. Parents are sensitive and sensible.

Table 4.073

Time given to response

Sufficient Time	No.
Yes	15
No	05

Sufficient time is given to response in 15cases, 05 of them didn't get sufficient time. Most of them take sufficient time to respond. Sufficient time is given to comprehend the matter.

Table 4.074

Motivates to do daily routine

Motivation	No.
Yes	14
No	04
No response	02

14 are motivated to do daily routine, 04 aren't, 02gives no response. High in number get motivated for their daily routine. Motivation always inspires the person to learn things, especially language.

Table 4.075

Experiences given for that purpose

Daily experiences	No.
To maintain house	13
Daily routine	08
Small repairing	05
Help in kitchen	08
Involved in function	13
All above	01
No exposure	01
No response	01

Experiences given for that purpose are as follows:13of them to maintain house,08 of them in daily routine,05 have chance in small repairing,08 of them help in kitchen,13 are involved in function,01 get all above mentioned experiences,   01have no exposure,01gives no response.

Explorations for house hold duties as well as involvement in family functions are the main instances for experience. Doing work with hands, actual experiences benefit the language development.

Table 4.076

Obstacles in experiences

Obstacles	No.
To know her feelings	01
To call someone	01

No response	18

01 parent cannot understand the feelings of their child, 01 child is unable to call someone, and 18 give no response. Most of them did not respond .No guess about obstacles.

Table 4.077

Environment around the child

Audible surroundings	No.
Yes	12
No	07
No response	01

12 children are always in environment having different sounds around them, 07 aren't, 01gives no response. Many of them are always in talkative surrounding. It can be motivational for deaf to learn language.

Table 4.078

Response for every new sound

Responses	No.
Yes	14
No	05
No response	01

14of them responds every new sound, 05don't, 01gives no response. Many of them are eager to respond every new sound. They carry listening capacity of different sounds.

Table 4.079

Response to differentiation of sound

Speaks about differentiation	No.
Yes	09
No	10

No response	01

09of them speaks about differentiation in sound, 10 don't, 01gives no response. Many of them do not speak about the similarities and differences of sound. They are not able to recognize the similarities and differences of sound.

Table 4.080

Parent's response about differentiation of sound

Speaks about differentiation	No.
Yes	11
No	07
No response	02

11 parents speak about the similarities and differences of sound with their child, 07 don't, and 02 of them give no response. Many of the parents speak about the similarities and differences of sound. Pronunciation differs the meaning of the words.

Table 4.081

Frequency of responses to the outer sounds

Frequency of responses	No.
Yes	12
No	07
No response	01

12 of them responds continuously the outer sounds, 07, don't, 01gives no response. Most of them are frequently responses to the outer sound. It is an important stage in learning language.

Table 4.082

Tendency to respond the sounds in the house

Responses in house increased	No.
Yes	13

No	06
No response	01

13children have their tendency increased to respond the sounds in the house, 06don't, 01gives no response. Most of them have increasing tendency to respond the sounds at home. Important stage of informal conversation is increase in tendency to respond the sounds in the house

Table 4.083

Production of sound

Creation of sound	No.
Yes	16
No	04

16 children create sounds on their own, 04 don't create any sound. Many of them like to produce some kind of noise. This is effort to speak, try to communicate with other person.

Table 4.084

Easiest way of comprehension

Way of communication	No.
Listening	02
Seeing	14
Talking	05
Tactile	03
No response	03

02 of them find listening as easiest way to comprehend the words, 14 find seeing, 05 find talking, 03 find tactile, 03 gives no response. For comprehension, visual is the easiest way. It's their best learning style.

Table 4.085

Quality of reading skill

Quality of loud reading	No.
Low	13
Moderate	01
Good	04
No response	02

13 of them have low quality of loud reading, 01 have moderate quality, 04 have good quality, 02gives no response. Most of them have comparatively low quality of loud reading, than normal children.

Table 4.086

Difficulty while reading

Difficulty in reading	No.
Yes	16
No	02
No response	02

16 of them experiences difficulty in reading, 02didn't, 02gives no response. Reading is very difficult task for majority of them. Reading and speech is not very easy.

Table 4.087

Types of difficulties in reading

Types of difficulty	No.
Lip movement	01
Reading not understandable	01
Cannot pronounce	01
Stammering	01

Wrong reading method	01
No response	15

Types of difficulty are as follows: 01 in lip movement, 01 whose reading is not understandable, 01while pronunciation, 01 get stammering, 01 develop wrong reading method, 15gives no response. Awkward lip movements, reading not understandable, wrong reading method, incorrect pronunciation are some of the reading difficulties. Main causes and effects of reading difficulties.

Table 4.088

Face reading of speaker's face

Continuous look	No.
Yes	18
No	02

18 of them look constantly to speaker's face, 02 don't. Most of them stare at speaker's face during conversation. Try to continue converse without break.

Table 4.089

Eye contact with speaker

Constant eye contact	No.
Yes	12
No	08

12 of them keep eye contact consistently, 08 don't keep eye contact. Most of them maintain eye contact with speaker constantly. Essential condition for every hearing impaired.

Table 4.090

Imitation of the gestures of speaker

Imitation	No.
Yes	18

No	02

18 of them imitates the gestures of speaker, 02 don't imitate. Most of them are habitual to imitate the gestures of the speaker. Sometimes imitation of actions leads to process of understanding.

Table 4.091

Responds spontaneously with sound

Responses	No.
Yes	13
No	06
No response	01

13 children responds spontaneously with sound, 06 didn't respond, 01gives no response. Many of them respond spontaneously with sound. Have opportunity of respond to stimuli.

Table 4.092

Use of humming

Use of humming	No.
Yes	08
No	10
No response	02

08children uses humming, 10 don't use humming, 02gives no response. A few of them have natural humming. It is a natural tendency to keep one happy.

Table 4.093

Uses the consonants and vowels having less and more time span

Use of words	No.
Yes	07
No	10

No response	03

07 of them use the consonants and vowels having less and more time span, 10don't, 03 gives no response. Very few of them use the consonants and vowels having less and more time span. This is a stage in process of learning grammar.

Table 4.094

Span of speech

Speech span	No.
Yes	01
No	16
No response	03

Only one child has good span of speech, 16 don't have, 03gives no response. Most of them are not eager to make speech of less and more time span. This is in process of self talk.

Table 4.095

Span of dialogue

Dialogue span	No.
Yes	03
No	14
No response	03

03 of them have dialogue of less and more time span, 14 don't have, 03No response. Most of them do not have dialogues of less and more time span. Ready for conversation and take opportunity.

Table 4.096

Control o breathing while speaking

Quality of breathing	No.
Yes	13

No	04
No response	03

13 carries good, controlled breathing while speaking, 04cannot control, 03gives no response. Most of them have good, controlled breathing while speaking. Control over exhaling and emotions, while talking.

Table 4.097

Obstacles during speech

Occurance of obstacles	No.
Yes	14
No	02
No response	04

14children experiences obstacles during speech, 02 don't experience obstacles, 04gives no response. Many of them experiences obstacles during speech. Types of obstacles are detected.

Table 4.098

Reaction while calling his/her name

Responds	No.
Yes	11
No	08
No response	01

11 of them responds every time while calling his/her name, 08 don't, 01gives no response. Many of them respond every time while calling his/her name. It is natural feeling of self introduction.

Table 4.099

Action instead of words during dialogue

Symbols instead of words	No.

Do gestures	05
Hand gestures	02
Signs	15
Writing	01

05 of them uses gestures instead of words during dialogue, 02 of them uses hand gestures instead of words during dialogue ,15 uses signs,01 expresses himself in written form. Most of the time signs are used instead of words during conversation. Try to keep dialogue without break.

Table 4.100

Movements/gestures for correct response

Accuracy	No.
Yes	17
No	01
No response	02

17 make accurate movement to response, 01 doesn't have accuracy, 02gives no response. Most of them make correct movements/gestures for correct response. Try to continue conversation through every available media.

Table 4.101

Expression for reaction

Oral response	No.
Yes	08
No	11
No response	01

08 of them try continuous oral responses, 11 don't try, 01gives no response. Many of them do not make sound for correct responses. It means not interested to continue conversation or try to find the right action.

Table 4.102

Action response

Try to communicate	No.
Yes	12
No	04
No response	04

12 of them try to communicate through their behaviour, 04 don't try, 04gives no response. Many of them try to communicate through their behaviour. Most of the time non-verbal communication is highly impressive and appreciated.

Table 4.103

Length of the sentences

Use one/two worded sentences	No.
Yes	08
No	12

08 speak the sentences having one/two words, 12 don't speak. Few of them speak the sentences having one/two words. Try to speak grammatically correct.

Table 4.104

Answers to the questions like where, when, what, why

Thoughtful responses	No.
e.g. article	09
Person	12
Picture	08
Incidence	07
Yes	14

No	03
No response	01

09 of them answers curiously about article, 12 about person,08 about picture,07 about incidence,14 answers to the wh- type questions,03 don't answer,01gives no response. Many of them answers curiously, thoughtfully to the questions like where, when, what, why about the articles and persons. They try to improve verbal ability with logical thinking.

Table 4.105

Use of various books by parents

Use of books	No.
Yes	04
No	15
No response	01

04 parents use various books for language development, 15 don't use any, 01gives no response. Very few parents use various types of books for language development. This shows parent's readiness to keep their child update.

Table 4.106

Involvement of parents in School activities

Parent's involvement	No.
Yes	14
No	04
No response	02

14 parents participate in school activities, 04 don't participate, 02gives no response. Parents are involved in group activities with their children. This is building awareness of parents with school activities and logical behaviour accordingly.

Table 4.107

Attendance to Conduction of workshops

149

Attend workshops	No.
Yes	14
No	04
No response	02

14 parents attend workshops conducted by school, 04 don't attend, 02gives no response. Many of them attend workshops conducted by schools. This shows active participation of parents in language development.

Table 4.108

Co-operation with teachers and speech trainer

Co-operation	No.
Yes	18
No	02

18 children co-operates with teachers and speech trainer, 02 don't co-operate. Many of them co-operates with teachers and speech trainers. Necessary action is taken for speech and language development.

Table 4.109

Use of guidance

Guidance is useful	No.
Yes	16
No	01
No response	03

16children are facilitate by teacher's guidance, 01don't get facilitate, 03gives no response. The guidance of teachers and speech trainers is useful for many parents. Cross checking of results and effects.

Table 4.110

Reason behind usefulness

Way in use of	No.
Linguistic	09
Speech	05
Behaviour	10
No response	05

09 children have advantage in linguistic, 05 in speech, 10 in behaviour, 05 gives no response.
Many of them experiences behavioural change in their children, realising cause and effect.

Table 4.111

Obstacles during their guidance

Obstacle in guidance	No.
Yes	07
No	08
No response	05

07experiences obstacles during guidance, 08 don't experiences, 05gives no response. Few of
them experiences obstacle in guidance, accepting obstacles and find the way out.

Table 4.112

Persons help in language development

Persons who helps	No.
Friends	10
Parents	13
Teacher	17
Speech trainer	08

Relatives	05
No response	02

10 of them get help in language development by friends,13 by parents,17 by teachers,08 by speech trainer,05 by relatives,02gives no response. Teachers, parents and friends are most influential persons in language development. Language develops in formal and informal manner.

Table 4.113

Sufficient time for practice and guidance

Sufficient time for practice and guidance	No.
Yes	15
No	03
No response	02

15of them get sufficient time for practice and guidance, 03 of them don't have time, 02gives no response. Most of them get sufficient practice and guidance for language and language development. Convince the thought of guidance and give sufficient time to complete the language development process.

Table 4.114

Involvement of parents

Involvement	No.
Yes	15
No	05

15 parents are involved in language development, 05 don't get involved. Involvement of parents is high in number. Active participation of parents is valuable for development of child and her language.

Table 4.115

Difficulties in language and speech development

Type of difficulties	No.
Home work	02
Conversation at home	01
Can't understand child's speech	06
Repetition	01
Communication through signs	02
Use of aid	01
Purchasing an article in the shop	01
To convey our thoughts to the child	01
To convey through conversation	05
No response	09

Following are main difficulties find in language and speech development of hearing impaired:

02 parents find in home work,01 in conversation at home,06 can't understand child's speech,01 in repetition,02 in communication through signs, 01 in use of aid, 01in purchasing an article in the shop,01 to convey his thoughts to the child,05 to convey through conversation,09 gives no response.(1)To convey through conversation and (2) child's speech is not understandable are two major difficulties in language and speech development. It reflects the types of difficulties are varied and there is no readymade single solution to solve them.

4.03) Analysis of Data obtained by Experiment:

Researcher wanted to understand effect of independent variable that is 'Improvisation technique' on dependent variable that is 'language development of student having moderate and severe hearing loss.' This technique is used as an intervention for Experimental group for helping them in the language development. There are seven principles of improvisation: trust, acceptance, attentive listening, spontaneity, storytelling, nonverbal communication, warm-ups.

Improvisation is used as a Teaching Technique for students to construct trust, support teamwork, improve communication and presentation skills,develop creative problem solving, react alertly and decisively to unexpected challenges, expand their comfort level with change and make their mind to encourage a supportive, improvisational philosophy.

Researcher conducted the activities everyday 90 minutes for 16 days through which the students need to learn how to adapt, adjust, listen, observe, agree, support, trust, and think fast.The inclusion of improvisation as a teaching strategy provides an excellent opportunity to teach students these necessary skills, as they increase in their abilities to achieve academic and professional success.

The tool used for the experimental method for pretesting and posttesting purpose was Educational progress test i.e. baseline test made by Government of Maharashtra (Maharashtra Pradhikaran Parishad, 2017). The 't' statistics was used to determine if there was any significant difference in the pre test and post test scores of base line test in Experimental group & Control group comparing for Writing+Vocabulary scores,Comprehension scores, Total scores. It presents testing of hypotheses and its interpretation. It also observes the graphical interpretation of the scores of experimental and control group and the discussion of the results.

A) Analysis of data obtained from the Experimental Group:

The data was analysed for Writing + Vocabulary scores, Comprehension scores, Total scores.

Table 4.116:

Pre and Post test scores for Writing + Vocabulary of Experimental group

Sr. No.	Pre	Post	Sr. No.	Pre	Post
1	15	15	12	9	9
2	15	15	13	5	5
3	15	15	14	5	5
4	15	15	15	5	5
5	15	15	16	5	5
6	15	15	17	5	5
7	15	15	18	5	5
8	9	10	19	5	5

9	8	10	20Graph	5	5
10	9	9	21	5	5
11	9	10			

Graph 4.1

Graph 4.1

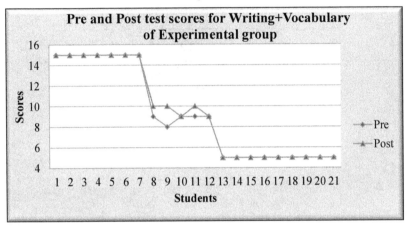

The line graph 4.1 suggests that there is a positive difference in Pre Post scores for Writing + Vocabulary in scores of 3 students out of 21 from Experimental group. In experimental group there are 5 girls and 2 boys of Std. 1(Total 7), 5 boys of Std. 2 (Total 5), 5 girls and 4 boys of Std.3 (Total 9).There are 10 girls and 11 boys in this group.3 students having positive change are boys from Std 2. All 10 girls and 8 boys of Std.s 1, 2, 3 show no change in their Pre and Post scores. All 7 students from Std. 1 got out of out scores in both Pre and Post tests. There is no evidence of negative change in scores.

Table 4.117

Pre and Post scores of Comprehension of Experimental Group

Sr. No.	Pre	Post	Sr. No.	Pre	Post
1	0	0	12	1	1
2	0	0	13	1	5
3	0	0	14	4	6
4	0	0	15	4	5
5	0	0	16	2	0

6	0	0	17	1	2
7	0	0	18	2	4
8	1	0	19	0	0
9	1	5	20	2	1
10	1	1	21	1	4
11	3	2			

Graph 4.2

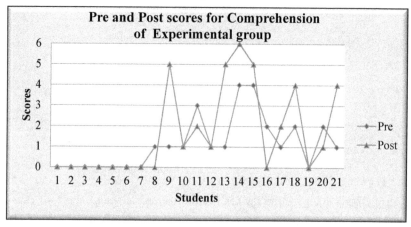

The line graph 4.2 suggests that there seems a positive difference in Pre Post scores for Comprehension in scores of 7 students out of 21from Experimental group. In experimental group there are 5 girls and 2 boys of Std. 1(Total 7), 5 boys of Std. 2 (Total 5), 5 girls and 4 boys of Std.3 (Total 9).There are 10 girls and 11 boys in this group. Students having positive change are 5 girls from Std.3and 2 boys (each from Stds.2, 3). Students having negative change are 4 boys (2 each from Stds. 2, 3). Students having no change are 5 girls and 5 boys from Stds. 1, 2, 3 in their Pre and Post scores. All 7 students from Std. 1 scored zero in both Pre and Post tests.

Table 4.118

Pre and Post scores for Total of Experimental group

Sr. No.	Pre	Post	Sr. No.	Pre	Post
1	15	15	12	10	10
2	15	15	13	6	10

3	15	15	14	9	11
4	15	15	15	9	10
5	15	15	16	7	5
6	15	15	17	6	7
7	15	15	18	7	9
8	10	10	19	5	5
9	9	15	20	7	6
10	10	10	21	6	9
11	12	12			

Graph 4.3

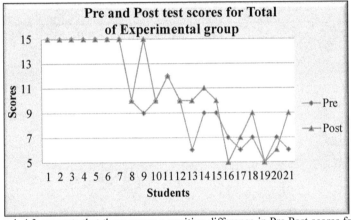

The line graph 4.3 suggests that there seems a positive difference in Pre Post scores for Total for 7 students out of 21from Experimental group. In experimental group there are 5 girls and 2 boys of Std. 1(Total 7), 5 boys of Std. 2 (Total 5), 5 girls and 4 boys of Std.3 (Total 9).There are 10 girls and 11 boys in this group.7 students having positive change are 5 girls from Std.3 and each 1 boy from Std 2, 3.Students having negative change are 2 boys from Std. 2. All 7 students from Std.1and 5 boys of Std.s 2, 3 show no change in their Pre and Post scores. All 7 students from Std. 1 got out of out scores in both Pre and Post tests.

B) Analysis of data obtained from the Control Group:

The data was analysed for Writing + Vocabulary scores,   Comprehension scores, Total scores

Table4.119:

Pre and Post scores for Writing + Vocabulary of Control group

Sr. No.	Pre	Post	Sr. No.	Pre	Post
1	15	15	11	5	5
2	8	7	12	5	5
3	8	7	13	5	10
4	6	6	14	5	5
5	7	6	15	5	5
6	8	7	16	5	5
7	8	10	17	5	5
8	9	6	18	5	5
9	9	5	19	4	5
10	5	5			

Graph 4.4

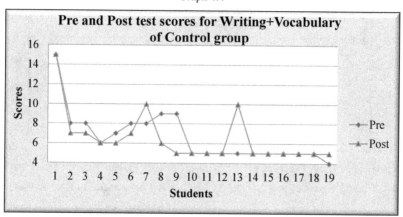

The line graph 4.4 suggests that there seems negative difference in Pre Post scores for Writing + Vocabulary for7students out of 19from Control group. In control group there is 1 boy of Std. 1(Total 1), 1 girl and 7 boys of Std. 2 (Total 8), 6 girls and 4 boys of Std.3 (Total 10).There are 7 girls and 12 boys in this group.2 students having positive change are boys from Std 2, 3. Students having negative change are 1 boy from Std.1 and6 girls from Stds.2, 3.6 girls and 4 boys of Std.s

1, 2, 3 show no change in their Pre and Post scores. One student from Std. 1 got out of out scores in both Pre and Post tests.

Table 4.120

Pre & Post scores for Comprehension of Control Group

Sr. No.	Pre	Post	Sr. No.	Pre	Post
1	0	0	11	1	0
2	0	0	12	1	1
3	0	0	13	3	0
4	0	0	14	3	1
5	0	0	15	3	2
6	0	0	16	2	1
7	0	0	17	1	1
8	0	0	18	2	2
9	0	1	19	0	0
10	1	0			

Graph 4.5

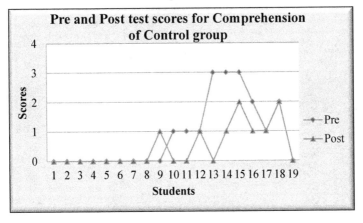

The line graph 4.5 suggests that there seems negative difference in Pre Post scores for Comprehension for 5 students out of 19from Control group. In control group there is 1 boy of Std. 1(Total 1), 1 girl and 7 boys of Std. 2 (Total 8), 6 girls and 4 boys of Std.3 (Total 10).There

159

are 7 girls and 12 boys in this group.6 students having negative change are 4 girls and 2 boys from Std.3. Students having positive change is 1 girl from Std.2 .2 girls and 10 boys of Std.s 1, 2, 3 show no change in their Pre and Post scores. One student from Std. 1 scored zero in both Pre and Post tests.

Table 4.121

Pre and Post scores for total of Control Group

Sr. No.	Pre	Post	Sr. No.	Pre	Post
1	15	15	11	6	5
2	8	7	12	6	6
3	8	7	13	8	10
4	6	6	14	8	6
5	7	6	15	8	7
6	8	7	16	7	6
7	8	10	17	6	6
8	9	6	18	7	7
9	9	6	19	4	5
10	6	5			

Graph 4.6

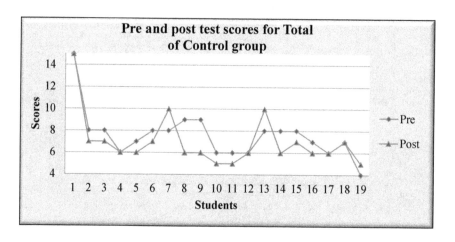

160

The line graph 4.6 suggests that there seems negative difference in Pre Post scores for Total 11 students out of 19from Control group. In control group there is 1 boy of Std. 1(Total 1), 1 girl and 7 boys of Std. 2 (Total 8), 6 girls and 4 boys of Std.3 (Total 10).There are 7 girls and 12 boys in this group.3 students having positive change are 1 girl from Std.2 and 2 boys from Std. 3. Students having negative change are 6 boys from Std.2 and 4 girls and 1 boy from Std.3.2 girls and 1 boy each from Std.s 1, 2, 3 show no change in their Pre and Post scores. One student from Std. 1 got out of out scores in both Pre and Post tests.

C) Analysis of data obtained from Comparison of (Post-Pre) scores between Experimental and Control Groups:

The data was analysed for (Post- Pre) scores of Writing + Vocabulary test, Comprehension test, and Total test.

Table 4.122

(Post-Pre) scores for Writing+Vocabulary of Experimental and Control groups

Sr. No.	Experimental Group	Control Group	Sr. No.	Experimental Group	Control Group
1	0	0	12	0	0
2	0	-1	13	0	5
3	0	-1	14	0	0
4	0	0	15	0	0
5	0	-1	16	0	0
6	0	-1	17	0	0
7	0	2	18	0	0
8	1	-3	19	0	1
9	2	-4	20	0	
10	0	0	21	0	
11	1	0			

Graph 4.7

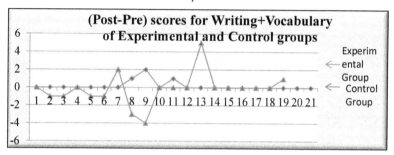

The graph 4.7 shows that the difference between Pre and Post is positive for Experimental Group and it is negative for Control Group. In Experimental group there are 10 girls and 11 boys i.e. total 21 students. In Control group there are 7 girls and 11 boys i.e. total 19 students. There are 10 students in Experimental group and 03 students in Control group having positive difference between Pre and Post tests. The number of scores in Experimental group is more than that of in Control group. There is no student in Experimental group and 14 students in Control group having negative difference between Pre and Post tests. The number of scores in Experimental group is very less than that of in Control group. There are 11students in Experimental group and 2 students in Control group having no change between Pre and Post tests. The number of scores in Experimental group is more than that of in Control group.

Table 4.123

(Post – Pre) for Comprehension of Experimental and Control Groups

Sr. No.	Experimental Group	Control Group	Sr. No.	Experimental Group	Control Group
1	0	0	12	0	0
2	0	0	13	4	-3
3	0	0	14	2	-2
4	0	0	15	1	-1
5	0	0	16	-2	-1
6	0	0	17	1	0
7	0	0	18	2	0
8	-1	0	19	0	0

9	4	1	20	-1	
10	0	-1	21	3	
11	-1	-1			

Graph 4.8

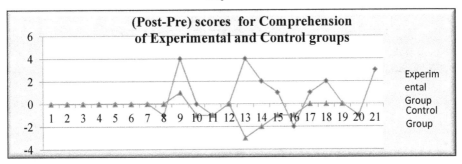

The graph 4.8 shows that the difference between Pre and Post is positive for Experimental Group and it is negative for Control Group. There are 7 students in Experimental group and 1 student in Control group having positive difference between Pre and Post tests. The number of scores in Experimental group is more than that of in Control group. There are 4 student in Experimental group and 6 students in Control group having negative difference between Pre and Post tests. The number of scores in Experimental group is less than that of in Control group. There are 10 students in Experimental group and 12 students in Control group having no change between Pre and Post tests. The number of scores in Experimental group is less than that of in Control group.

Table 4.124

(Post – Pre) for Total of Experimental & Control Groups

Sr. No.	Experimental Group	Control Group	Sr. No.	Experimental Group	Control Group
1	0	0	12	0	0
2	0	-1	13	4	2
3	0	-1	14	2	-2
4	0	0	15	1	-1
5	0	-1	16	-2	-1

6	0	-1	17	1	0
7	0	2	18	2	0
8	0	-3	19	0	1
9	6	-3	20	-1	
10	0	-1	21	3	
11	0	-1			

Graph 4.9

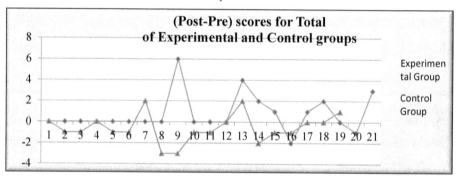

The graph 4.9 shows that the difference between Pre and Post is positive for Experimental Group and it is negative for Control Group. There are 7 students in Experimental group and 3 students in Control group having positive difference between Pre and Post tests. The number of scores in Experimental group is more than that of in Control group. There are 2 students in Experimental group and 11 students in Control group having negative difference between Pre and Post tests. The number of scores in Experimental group is very less than that of in Control group. There are 12 students in Experimental group and 5 students in Control group having no change between Pre and Post tests. The number of scores in Experimental group is more than that of in Control group.

4.04) Testing the Hypothesis:

This section provides results of analysis of research hypotheses applying 't' statistics.

The hypotheses are:

(1) There will be significant difference in pre test and post test scores for language development in the experimental group.

(2)There will be no significant difference in pre test and post test scores for language development in the control group..

(3)There will be a positive gain in the language development of experimental group as compared to that in control group.

A) Research Hypothesis 1

There will be significant difference in pre test and post test scores for language development in the experimental group.

The null hypothesis (H_0):

There will be no significant difference in pre test and post test scores for language development in the experimental group.

The alternative hypothesis (H_a):

Post test scores for language development will be greater than the pre test scores in the experimental group

As the hypothesis is unidirectional, one tailed t test was used for the statistical analysis with confidence level of 0.05%

Table 4.125

't' statistics for Hypothesis 1

		Paired Differences			t	df	P value
		Mean	Std. Deviation	Std. Error Mean			
Writing+ Vocabulary	Post-Pre	0.19	0.51	0.11	-1.71	20	.104
Comprehension	Post-Pre	0.57	1.60	0.35	-1.64	20	.117
Total	Post-Pre	0.76	1.79	0.39	-1.95	20	.065
a. Groups = Experimental Group							

Since p value > 0.05 at significance level, there is no sufficient evidence to reject the null hypothesis. We accept null hypothesis.

Hence, there is no significant difference in pre test and post test scores for language development in the experimental group.

B) Research Hypothesis 2

There will be no significant difference in pre test and post test scores for language development in the control group.

The null hypothesis (H_0):

There will be no significant difference in pre test and post test scores for language development in the control group.

The alternative hypothesis (H_a):

There will be significant difference in pre test and post test scores for language development in the control group.

As the hypothesis is non directional hypothesis, two tailed t test was used for the statistical analysis with confidence level of 0.05%

Table 4.126

't' statistics for Hypothesis 2

		Paired Differences			t	df	P value
		Mean	Std. Deviation	Std. Error Mean			
Pair 1	Post-Pre	-0.15	1.80	0.41	0.38	18	.707
Pair 2	Post-Pre	-0.42	0.90	0.21	2.04	18	.057
Pair 3	Post-Pre	-0.58	1.35	0.31	1.87	18	.077
a. Groups = Control Group							

Since p value > 0.05 at significance level, there is no sufficient evidence to reject the null hypothesis. We accept null hypothesis.

Hence, there is no significant difference in pre test and post test scores for language development in the control group.

C) Research Hypothesis 3

There will be a positive gain in the language development of experimental group as compared to that in control group.

The null hypothesis (H₀):

There will be no positive gain in the language development of experimental group as compared to that in control group.

The alternative hypothesis (Hₐ):

There will be a positive gain in the language development of experimental group as compared to that in control group.

The test used is t test for two independent samples.

Table 4.127

't' statistics for Hypothesis 3

		Levene's Test for Equality of Variances		t-test for Equality of Means		
		F	Sig.	t	df	P value
Writing+Vocabulary	Equal variances assumed	5.041	.031	.849	38	.401
	Equal variances not assumed			.813	20.621	.425
Comprehension	Equal variances assumed	4.743	.036	2.383	38	.022
	Equal variances not assumed			2.447	32.117	.020
Total	Equal variances assumed	.759	.389	2.658	38	.011

167

	Equal variances not assumed			2.696	36.857	.011
Gain Score	Equal variances assumed	.472	.496	2.627	38	.012
	Equal variances not assumed			2.659	37.246	.011

Since p value < 0.05 at significance level, there is sufficient evidence to reject the null hypothesis. We accept the alternative hypothesis.

Hence, there is a positive gain in the language development of experimental group as compared to that in control group.

INDEX

CHAPTER 5: Discussion and Conclusions

5.00) Introduction   170

5.01) Findings of the Survey: a) By the teachers, b) By the parents   170

5.02) Findings of the Experiment   173

5.03) Conclusions: 174

A) Conclusions of the Survey: a) By the teachers, b) By the parents   175

B) Conclusions of the Experiment   177

5.05)Findings from Interviews of : a)the teacher educators, b) parents   178

5.06)Suggestions from : a)the teacher educators ,b) parents   181

5.07) Observations after implementation of the Experiment   182

5.08) Discussions of the results   183

A) Possible Reasons for finding Non -significant difference for   the   183
Experimental group in the posttest

B) Possible Reasons for finding negative difference for the Control group in   183
the posttest

Introduction:

In chapter 4 the analysis of data obtained by Survey and the statistical procedures of the experiment were described.

This chapter reveals findings of the Survey and the Experiment. It also describes conclusions of the Survey and conclusions after testing the hypotheses of the experiment. Reasons for finding non -significant difference for the Experimental group in the posttest and reasons for finding negative difference for the Control group in the posttest are also discussed in this chapter.

Findings of the Survey:

a) The analysis of the data for the survey from teachers reveals that:

1) Following are the difficulties in language development of hearing impaired child:

1. Make signs/acts instead of words during dialogue. Most of them cannot speak the sentences having one/two words.

2. Most children have poor level of vocabulary.

2) The reasons behind the difficulties in language development of hearing impaired are:

1. Most of the students have hearing loss more than 61dB, i.e. moderately severe and severe loss.

2. Very less among them tests the hearing loss frequently. Early intervention may benefit the language development.

3. Most of the children have conductive hearing loss, where hearing aid may help in limit. Sensory-neural hearing loss is not curable and repairable.

4. Most of the children have moderate or severe hearing loss. There is residual hearing according to hearing impairment which results into possible language development.

3) The present ways and methods applied by teachers to overcome these difficulties are:

1. There is awareness of using advanced technology in teaching learning process. High tech equipments are used with appropriate hearing loss. The basic necessities of hearing impaired are fulfilled with these equipments.

2. Most of the teachers experiences that the learning material is useful for other students also, when used by their colleagues, indicates the validity and reliability of the material.

3. All students uses hearing aid.

4. Workshops are meant to enrich the parents in new knowledge and technology.

5. Most of the children were immediately supported by the hearing aid after diagnosis. Acceptance of impairment and remedial action had been taken immediately by parents.

6. The school record in the form of progress card is supposed to be the main mode of child's record. Language development of a child shows the involvement of parents, teachers, and environment.

7. Many of them are eager to respond every new sound. They carry listening capacity of different sounds.

8. Most of them are frequently responds to the outer sound. It is an important stage in learning language.

4) The processes which are important for language development of hearing impaired:

1. Most of the children were immediately supported by the hearing aid after diagnosis. Acceptance of impairment and remedial action had been taken immediately by parents.

3. Most of the children are tested by experts. This shows the authenticity in early years.

4. Reports of the correct diagnosis of all the children were confirmed by the expert.

5. Many of them can maintain the hearing aid regularly. They realises the need and importance of the equipment.

6. Behind the ear hearing aid is widely used by the children, suitable device according to diagnosis.

b) The analysis of the data for the survey from parents reveals that:

1) Following are the difficulties in language development of hearing impaired child:

1. Do not have sufficient vocabulary for daily routine.

2. Reading is very difficult task for majority of them. Reading and speech is not very easy.

2) The reasons behind the difficulties in language development of hearing impaired are:

1. Most of the family members are passed from secondary school.

2. The parents are from very low income group. The status of most of the families has very low socio-economic background.

3. Most of the children have hearing loss in both the ears. Parents confirm the information about deafness.

3) The present ways and methods applied by parents to overcome these difficulties are:

1. In spite of their deafness most of the children are treated as a normal child. They are not overprotected. Parents are sensitive and sensible.

2. Most of them stare at speaker's face during conversation. Try to continue converse without break.

3. Most of them maintain eye contact with speaker constantly. Essential condition for every hearing impaired.

4. Most of them are habitual to imitate the gestures of the speaker. Sometimes imitation of actions leads to process of understanding.

5. Many of them attend workshops conducted by schools. This shows active participation of parents in language development.

6. Parents are involved in group activities with their children. This is building awareness of parents with school activities and logical behaviour accordingly.

7. Many of them co-operates with teachers and speech trainers. Necessary action is taken for speech and language development.

4) The processes which are important for language development of hearing impaired:

1. Most of the parents diagnosed the hearing loss before the 3rd year, which is a critical period for language development. This is very valuable period for developing and learning any language.

2. Hearing aid is used consistently by majority of children, possibly benefits more.

3. Many children are trained to take care of hearing aid. Child realises importance of the device. Child is aware of how and why it is to be handled carefully.

4. Many parents have interaction with other parents. Hence they get more information other than their knowledge.

5. Most of the parents keep the records of responses given by their child. The change in responses leads to change in practice.

Findings of the experiment:

1) There is a less in number of students in post test scores having better performance In Writing+ Vocabulary , the number of students having better performance in Comprehension than in Writing + Vocabulary is more but the number of students having better performance overall for Experimental group is very less which shows that the programme is found to be less effective.

Since p value > 0.05 at significance level, there is no sufficient evidence to reject the null hypothesis. We accept null hypothesis.

Hence, there is no significant difference in pre test and post test scores for language development in the experimental group.

2) There is reduction in number of students having better performance in post test, the number of students showing poor performance in Comprehension is decreased as compared to Writing + Vocabulary posttest ,the number of students showing poor performance overall in post test increased for the Control group.

Since p value > 0.05 at significance level, there is no sufficient evidence to reject the null hypothesis. We accept null hypothesis.

Hence, there is no significant difference in pre test and post test scores for language development in the control group.

3) The difference between Pre and Post is positive for Experimental Group and it is negative for Control Group in overall performance. It implies that the scores are increased from Pre to Post for Experimental Group and scores are decreased from Pre to Post for Control Group.

Since p value < 0.05 at significance level, there is sufficient evidence to reject the null hypothesis. We accept the alternative hypothesis.

Hence, there is a positive gain in the language development of experimental group as compared to that in control group.

Conclusions:

A) Conclusions of the Survey:

a) The data for the survey from teachers reveals that:

1) Following are the difficulties in language development of hearing impaired child:

Quality of reading skill of most of the students is very poor. They have difficulties while reading, like wrong lip movement, reading not understandable, cannot pronounce properly, stammering, wrong reading method etc.

2) The reasons behind the difficulties in language development of hearing impaired are:

1. Sufficient time for the language development is not given from the family members.

2. There is a misconception that, if there is no speech, there is no language.

3) The present ways and methods applied by teachers and parents to overcome these difficulties are:

1. Use of various visual aids while teaching and interaction among teachers of various grades take place in a large scale.

2. There is a wide range of the sources used by the teachers for language learning other than books.The teachers are user friendly with new technology and experienced in advance technology. Variation in sources builds the base of the thought in language development of the children. This shows the variation in activities for language development.Activities like picture medium, dramatization, learn through play, make words incline to raise the vocabulary.

3. Sufficient time is given to comprehend the matter.

4. Control over exhaling and emotions, while talking.

4) The processes which are important for language development of hearing impaired:

1. The audiometry.

2. Analysis of audiometry and its results.

3. The non-verbal communication is highly impressive and appreciated.

4. Deciding remedies as per need.

5. Plan of action considering hearing loss

b) The data for the survey from the parents reveals that:

1) Following are the difficulties in language development of hearing impaired child:

1. There are difficulties in language and speech development like- completing home work, conversation at home, can't understand child's speech, repetition, communication through signs, use of aid, purchasing an article from the shop, to convey our thoughts to the child, to convey through conversation etc.

2. They have comparatively low quality of loud reading, than normal children.

2) The reasons behind the difficulties in language development of hearing impaired are:

1. Parents are unaware that children learn language on their own.

2. Inconsistency in follow-up for language development is observed.

3. Most of the mechanical sounds are audible than human voice to the hearing impaired children.

3) The present ways and methods applied by teachers and parents to overcome these difficulties are:

1. Parents are aware of different ways, techniques or technology other than in our country.

2. Members at home keep the environment free to speak and learn.

3. There is talkative, simple and safe surrounding at home.

4. Important stage of informal conversation is increase in tendency to respond the sounds in the house.

4) The processes which are important for language development of hearing impaired:

1. Parents are early aware of the deafness.

2. The deafness was accepted by parents.

3. Spends extra time and more efforts to language development.

4. Experiences constant explorations for house hold duties as well as involvement in family functions.

B) Conclusions of the Experiment:

(1) There is no significant difference in pre test and post test scores for language development in the experimental group.

(2) There is no significant difference in pre test and post test scores for language development in the control group.

(3) There is a positive gain in the language development of experimental group as compared to that in control group, after the implementation of the programme.

This implies the improvisation technique was found to be effective in the language development of the hearing impaired children.

As Training Program was conducted with Experimental group, they were inclined towards giving objective answers; whereas Control group may not answer in objective manner.

Though the posttest score was not significant for the Experimental group, there is a gain for the Experimental group than the Control group. This is because there are 2 students out of 21 in Experimental group and 11 students out of 19 in Control group having negative difference between Pre and Post tests. The number of scores in Experimental group is very less than that of in Control group. The difference between Pre and Post is more positive for Experimental Group and it is more negative for Control Group.

5.04 A) Findings from Interviews of

a) the teacher educators

From the findings, the greatest difficulty for students with Hearing Impairment in writing construction was the adequate vocabulary as stated by most teachers. This was also noted in the performance of students in the given tests. The writing of the essay was about how many words the reader had acquired to organize the facts and to reflect on the subject on which he was to write. Without adequate vocabulary it was difficult to write the make-up as it was necessary for their complexity. A deaf child has a tendency to use Sign Language structures instead of Marathi language frameworks when writing songs. Other challenges include illiteracy, poor spelling, abandonment, regression and substitution.

Hearing impaired face challenges in terms of abnormal cognitive skills, poor memory skills, inability to read fluently, inadequate vocabulary and limited cognitive skills.

In addition to the limitations of inclusion, the very complexity of the task of learning a language with a highly restricted knowledge can lead to a loss of motivation. Another paradox is the language barriers and the fact that the deaf community uses visual language, Sign Language, which deaf people acquire without effort and that offer a focus on cultural unity. Attitude towards SL is as complex in its knowledge as a minor language in most disciplines, its general language influencing it to some degree. The attitude towards Marathi is complicated by the fact that learning Marathi is determined by a hearing-driven educational institution and that SL is not used as a language of instruction.

Hearing loss can have a profound effect on a child's D / HH behavior and self-esteem. Students may find themselves different if they have hearing or communication problems, especially if they wear cochlear accessories / hearing aids and / or use an FM system (wireless communication). Reduced communication power can interfere with the development of appropriate social skills. This negative image can recur if an inexperienced teacher makes a mistake to a D / HH child "by dreaming," or "hearing when he wants to," or "not trying." In addition to the aforementioned effects, many hearing-impaired children may be more apathetic, easily frustrated, and less confident in the classroom than their hearing-impaired peers. The following is a summary of the reasons for learning failure:

1. Workshops shot once and wide but do not work.

2. Topics are often chosen by people other than those offered in-service.

3. Follow-up support for ideas and practices presented during in-service programs takes place in very small cases.

4. Follow-up testing occurs rarely.

5. Workplace programs do not usually address individual needs and participants' concerns.

6. Most programs include teachers from many different schools and / or school districts, but there is no recognition of the different effects of positive and negative within the program to which they should return.

7. There is a serious lack of any basis for the planning and implementation of internal work plans that will ensure their effective implementation.

b) Findings from Interviews of parents:

Deaf children often find it difficult to learn their parents' language, in many cases hearing it. The main reason for these problems is the limited language input that reaches children: Loss of hearing alone serves as a powerful filter for language data, as well as information obtained from residual listening, as well as visual sources such as lip-reading and sign language presentations.

Deaf children of deaf parents can follow a variety of paths. This may depend more on parental characteristics, history, and environment than on the developmental process of hearing-impaired children. The developmental difficulties caused by hearing loss should be of great interest to ethical scientists and medical professionals alike, and it is clear that there are many issues that need to be addressed.

Often these children are more tired than their hearing peers because of the level of effort required listening during the day. Rising levels of fatigue put these students at risk for irritating behavior in the classroom. These factors can have a significant impact on their academic performance. With the right knowledge, teachers and professionals can play an active and supportive role in a child's D / HH life.

5.04 B) Suggestions have been given

a) by teacher educators to teach CWSN in general classes including: (Children with Special Needs)

1. Provision of school ramps

2. Secure structure

3. Suitable playground space (CWSN swing)

4. The need for clean water

5. Sanitation

6. The allotment of teacher teachers should be 1:20

7. Accommodation arrangements should be comfortable

8. One separate room for household chores

9. Provision of audio and visual aids

10. Provision of computer class

11. Public Awareness Camps

12. Resource teacher in all schools

13. Classrooms should be on the ground floor (CWSN)

14. A training program on CWSN strategies for in-service teachers should be conducted in the actual classrooms in order to obtain practical information regarding CWSN teaching in the classroom itself.

15. There should be Game corners in the school

16. It should be given to the teacher's assistant

17. Morning classes for classes for 1 to 5 and evening classes for 6 to 10 classes

18. The program must be under CWSN

19. Appropriate transport services should be provided to students

20. Monitor the learner otherwise getting low pass marks.

Examples of good practice suggested:-

a) Long essay type essay questions with short answer questions - this could be accompanied by viva in Sign Language (translator available).

b) Oral language tests are included in the written tests.

c) Written articles have been replaced by visual works.

d) Oral submissions have been replaced by signed submissions (present interpreters).

e) Some of the test material was signed to a video camera and translated by an interpreter rather than written.

b) Suggestions from Parents:

Start early for intervention.

Check out the options of different learning strategies.

Get the child to install hearing aids.

Talk to other parents.

Join a parent group, talk, and get help.

Keep the right to change your mind.

Stay aware for forever.

Take one task at a time.

Insist; don't give up, the rewards are worth it.

Relax! Don't forget to enjoy your child.

Live life to the fullest!

Observations after the implementation of the Experiment:

1. Ice braking games like wolf-goat, mirror image were conducted to interact each other and to form a homogeneous group. Every member of the experimental group developed the communication skill to construct trust and support teamwork.

2. Physical movements of own body parts lead to create awareness of own body, ready for knowing body language. Many of them try to communicate through signs and sign language.

3. Exercise like Mirror image helped in action and reaction to react alertly and decisively to unexpected challenges.

4. Believe in others exercise built self confidence as well as believe in others to express their feelings.

5. Theatrical games and team building exercises were executed to share thoughts with actions and signs.

6. Drawings on paper with colours for self expressions were drawn.

7. Improvising various incidents using mime helped to know the roles of professionals like a painter, a sculptor, a policeman.

8. A structured frame work – composition of an incident to suggest an incident with body language developed spontaneity and trust.

9. Enacting concrete incident improved communication with others and helped in comprehension through dialogue, property, music.

10. Theatrical games were organised to enact abstract images to express abstract concepts through actions like famine, freedom, loyalty.

11. Improvisation explored opportunities to discover new ideas, improve communication and presentation skills.

12. Role playing and warm-ups provided safe, secure environment.

13. Non verbal communication and storytelling lead to create a collaborative narrative that connects dialogue through story and developed creative problem solving.

14. If Training Program is introduced in the school infrastructure, students will get abundant opportunities to educate themselves about language development.

15. While studying for the preparation of the Training Program, the researcher came to know various interesting facets of language development

16. It was a challenging task to make the entire training program interesting, innovative as well as educative. Plenty of exercises, stories, and activities made participants to actively participate in the sessions.

17. For learning language early intervention helps in development. It can be taught at primary school level, with easy and activity-based training sessions.

18. Parents, teachers, audiologists, speech trainers and close family members should have good communication practices so as to develop the language.

The improvisation technique was found to be effective in the language development of the hearing impaired children.

Discussion of the Results:

A) Possible Reasons for finding Non -significant difference for the Experimental group in the posttest:

1) The test given was made for normal students as well as special need students.

2) No student gains an identical score on test given at different times.

3) Poor effort taken by the students in attempting descriptive type questions.

4) Some of them might have difficulty in understanding the question.

B) Possible Reasons for finding negative difference for the Control group in the posttest:

1) The test given was made for normal students as well as special need students.

2) No student gains an identical score on test given at different times.

3) Poor effort taken by the students in attempting descriptive type questions.

4) Some of them might have difficulty in understanding the question.

5) Fatigue due to time of the test, Sunday morning.

6) Students might have a tendency of low score in written examination.

7) In absence of their regular teacher, students might have felt uncomfortable.

INDEX

CHAPTER 6: Summary

6.01) Introduction   186

6.02) Statement of problem   186

6.03) Objectives of the study   186

6.04) Survey Related Major research questions   186

6.05) Experiment Related Hypotheses   187

6.06) Variables   187

6.07) Research Design   187

6.08) Improvisation technique   188

6.09) Sample   189

6.10) Selection of the Tool   189

6.11) Major conclusions of the Research   189

  A) Conclusions of the Survey   189

  B) Conclusions of the Experiment   192

6.12) Educational implications of the Study   192

6.13) Suggestions for Future Research   193

6.14) Summary   193

This chapter gives the brief summary of the research.

6.01) Introduction:

The use of Improvisation in learning experiences would reduce the hurdles in language development .It will accelerate the process of language learning is a guess .If is found correct it would bring in transformation in the teaching learning of hearing impaired students. This indicates the direction of the effective and efficient modification in instructional system of hearing impaired students. In the end, the language learning process would be facilitated and in turn would facilitate their entire learning.

6.02) Statement of problem

conducting a survey of the present methods of language teaching applied by teachers from special school and parents of hearing impaired students with a view to overcoming the difficulties in language development and applying the improvisation technique for language development of hearing impaired students from residential school and testing its effectiveness from Pune city and a suburb of Pune.

6.03) Objectives of the study:

(1) To investigate difficulties in language development faced by the hearing impaired students, their teachers and parents

(2)To examine the present ways and methods of language teaching applied by teachers from special school and parents of hearing impaired students with a view to overcoming the difficulties in language development.

(3) To develop the Improvisation programme for hearing impaired students.

(4) To test the effectiveness of improvisation technique in language development.

6.04) Survey Related Major research questions:

1) What are the difficulties in language development of hearing impaired child?

4) Which processes are important for language development of hearing impaired?

3) What are the present ways and methods applied by teachers and parents to overcome these difficulties?

2) Why do these difficulties occur?

6.05) Experiment Related Hypotheses:

(1) There will be significant difference in pre test and post test scores for language development in the experimental group.

(2)There will be no significant difference in in pre test and post test scores for language development in the control group.

(3)There will be a positive gain in the language development of experimental group as compared to that in control group.

6.06) Variables:

The following variables are found in the present study

Independent Variable- In this research study, 'Improvisation Technique' is considered as an independent variable as this technique is supposed to be responsible for bringing about change .

Dependent Variables – In this research study, 'language development of students having moderate loss and moderately severe loss' is considered as dependent variable as it is the outcome of the change brought about by introduction of an independent variable.

Extrinsic Variables- In this research study, 'School environment, teaching methods of the teachers, and interaction of students with other students and their parents, interaction of parents with School' are considered as extrinsic variables as the above mentioned factors may affect changes in on the dependent variables. These factors are not measured in the study, may increase or decrease the magnitude of the relationship between independent and dependent variables.

6.07) Research Design:

The researcher is going to test the effectiveness of the technique of Improvisation in language development of hearing impaired student. The programme was of 16 days, one and half hour per day. The programme was tried out experimentally to test its effectiveness. In order to test the effectiveness of the technique of Improvisation in language development, an examination with the existing ways of language development is a prerequisite. So the survey and the experimental both the methods are to be selected. In the survey, difficulties in language development faced by teachers and parents with their hearing impaired students were investigated. The present methods of language teaching applied by teachers were examined. The efforts taken by the parents of hearing impaired students with a view to overcoming the difficulties in language development were investigated. The important processes for language development of hearing impaired were observed.

The effectiveness of improvisation technique in language development of hearing impaired students was tested. The research design for the study was Pretest-Posttest control and experimental group design. Taking into consideration the spread of population of students with moderate hearing loss and moderately severe loss, the random selection of the sample for control and experiment will be difficult. So equivalent groups of students were selected and distributed for control and experimental treatment. These groups were selected by researcher as the required sample was from equal socio, economical and educational background.

6.08) Improvisation technique:
Improvisation is a stimulating teaching strategy which promotes cooperation, collaboration, self- control, goal-oriented learning also as emotional intelligence skills. Improvisation bridges the gap between printed-book dialogues and natural usage, and can also help to bridge an identical gap between the classroom and real world situations by providing insights into the way to handle difficult situations. Drama and songs, for instance, strengthen the bond between thought and expression in language, and offer good listening practice. If Improvisation is taken into account as pedagogies within the sense of being a part of the eclectic approach to teaching, then it can become a main aid within the acquisition of communicative   competence.   .
Improvisation activities facilitate the sort of language behavior that ought to cause fluency, and if it's accepted that the learners want to find out language so as to form themselves understood within the language, then, improvisation does indeed, further this end. One of the best advantages to be gained from the utilization of drama, songs and games is that students become more confident in their use of language by experiencing the language in operation. Improvisation encourages adaptability, fluency, and communicative competence.

It puts language into context, and by giving learners experience of success in real-life situations it should arm them confidently for tackling the planet outside the classroom. Improvisation encourages students to mobilize their vocabulary, answer grammatical and syntactical accuracy, and develop cultural and social awareness, and gain confidence and fluency. Through constant repetition of words and phrases, they become conversant in them and are ready to say them with increasing fluency by encouraging self- expression; drama, especially, motivates students to use language confidently and creatively[5]. Improvisation enables the students to flex their emotional, mental also as physical muscles during a safe and controlled setting.

6.09) Sample:

In Pune city area and its suburb, there are 12 special primary schools for 970 deaf students and 108 working teachers. There are 3 residential schools with 150 students, 6 nonresidential schools with 535 students and 3 schools having 285 resident and nonresident students.

Total 20 parents and 21 teachers participated in the survey.

For execution of experimental method total 40 students participated from two residential schools. In Experimental group 21 students and in Control group 19 students were selected.

6.10) Selection of the Tool:

To investigate difficulties in language development faced by the hearing impaired students, their teachers and parents and to examine the present ways and methods of language teaching applied by teachers and parents, the survey was conducted .The researcher use the questionnaire for the teachers and parents. Interviews were also conducted to fulfill the purpose.

There is no separate test to evaluate writing, vocabulary and comprehension of hearing impaired. Hence the researcher decided to use baseline test made by Government of Maharashtra (Maharashtra Pradhikaran Parishad, 2017) for the experimental method for pretesting and posttesting.(in appendix).It could be useful for comparing writing, vocabulary and comprehension with normal children in future.

6.11) Major conclusions of the Research:

A) Conclusions of the Survey: a) The data for the survey from teachers reveals that:

1) Following are the difficulties in language development of hearing impaired child:

Quality of reading skill of most of the students is very poor. They have difficulties while reading, like wrong lip movement, reading not understandable, cannot pronounce properly, stammering, wrong reading method etc.

2) The reasons behind the difficulties in language development of hearing impaired are:

1. Sufficient time for the language development is not given from the family members.

2. There is a misconception that, if there is no speech, there is no language.

3) The present ways and methods applied by teachers and parents to overcome these difficulties are:

1. Use of various visual aids while teaching and interaction among teachers of various grades take place in a large scale.

2. There is a wide range of the sources used by the teachers for language learning other than books.The teachers are user friendly with new technology and experienced in advance technology. Variation in sources builds the base of the thought in language development of the children. This shows the variation in activities for language development.Activities like picture medium, dramatization, learn through play, make words incline to raise the vocabulary.

3. Sufficient time is given to comprehend the matter.

4. Control over exhaling and emotions, while talking.

4) The processes which are important for language development of hearing impaired:

1. The audiometry.

2. Analysis of audiometry and its results.

3. The non-verbal communication is highly impressive and appreciated.

4. Deciding remedies as per need.

5. Plan of action considering hearing loss

a) The data for the survey from the parents reveals that:

1) Following are the difficulties in language development of hearing impaired child:

1. There are difficulties in language and speech development like- completing home work, conversation at home, can't understand child's speech, repetition, communication through signs, use of aid, purchasing an article from the shop, to convey our thoughts to the child, to convey through conversation etc.

2. They have comparatively low quality of loud reading, than normal children.

2) The reasons behind the difficulties in language development of hearing impaired are:

1. Parents are unaware that children learn language on their own.

2. Inconsistency in follow-up for language development is observed.

3. Most of the mechanical sounds are audible than human voice to the hearing impaired children.

3) The present ways and methods applied by teachers and parents to overcome these difficulties are:

1. Parents are aware of different ways, techniques or technology other than in our country.

2. Members at home keep the environment free to speak and learn.

3. There is talkative, simple and safe surrounding at home.

4. Important stage of informal conversation is increase in tendency to respond the sounds in the house.

4) The processes which are important for language development of hearing impaired:

1. Parents are early aware of the deafness.

2. The deafness was accepted by parents.

3. Spends extra time and more efforts to language development.

4. Experiences constant explorations for house hold duties as well as involvement in family functions.

B) Conclusions of the Experiment:

(1) There is no significant difference in pre test and post test scores for language development in the experimental group.

(2)There is no significant difference in pre test and post test scores for language development in the control group.

(3)There is a positive gain in the language development of experimental group as compared to that in control group, after the implementation of the programme.

This implies the improvisation technique was found to be effective in the language development of the hearing impaired children.

6.12) Educational implications of the Study:

Improvisation is especially observable as a form of socialization. Because here main emphasis is on social learning with communication is its base. Improvisation is a technique to improve communication skill of normal as well as special need children. It can widely use as effective technique for different types of special need persons as well as children of all ages.

6.13) Suggestions for Future Research:

Instructional experiences in oral-aural language can be arranged to develop speech, individually and in groups.

Improvisation can be used as an evaluation tool for other special need children, like sight challenged or the gifted.

The programmes for development of speech and writing can be crafted for the experiences beyond the books.

Workshops can be conducted for special educators and teachers on different modes of learning, creative writing etc.

The programmes for vocabulary development can be organised, based on text books and other books out of syllabus.

Other forms of dramatics can be experimented for language development, like role playing, creative dramatics and puppetry.

6.14) Summary:

This describes the summary of conclusions of research regarding objectives with respect to research questions and hypotheses.

Objectives of the study	Research question/Hypothesis	Sample size	Analysis	Conclusions
(1)To investigate difficulties faced by the hearing impaired students, their teachers and parents.	(1) What are the difficulties in language development of hearing impaired child?	20 parents 21 teachers	-------------	* reading quality very poor. *difficulties while reading, like: wrong lip movement, reading not understandable, cannot pronounce properly, stammering, wrong reading method etc. * difficulties in language and speech development like- completing home work, conversation at home, can't understand child's speech, repetition, communication through signs, use of aid, purchasing an article , to convey our thoughts to the child, to convey through conversation etc. * cannot uses the consonants and vowels having less and more time span. *Do not speak for less and

				more time span. * experiences obstacles during speech. *do not speak about the similarities and differences of sound. *low quality of loud reading.
	(2) Why do these difficulties occur?	20 Parents 21 teachers	-------------	* only mother is involved in language development * Parents do not respond to obstacles. * A misconception: if there is no speech, there is no language. *children learn language on their own. *parents did not respond about reason of obstacles in contacts. *no follow-up is observed. * The mechanical sounds are audible than human voice. *less supportive for language development.
(2)To examine the present ways and methods of language	3) What are the present ways and methods applied by teachers and parents	20 Parents 21 Teachers	-------------	* co-operative nature of the teacher * eagerness to trying on different levels * Readiness to

teaching applied by teachers from special school and parents of hearing impaired students with a view to overcoming the difficulties in language development.	to overcome these difficulties?			experimentation. * understand the audiogram , aware of residual hearing * can prepare need based learning material. * Child spent more time with parents. * Parents aware of different ways, techniques or technology * Large range of the resources used by the teachers other than books. * user friendly with new technology * experienced in advance technology. * Variation in activities for language development. *Activities to raise the vocabulary. * aware of extra efforts to be taken for language development * tries to achieve the landmarks of the language development. *communicate face to face * feel free to talk at home. * have opportunity to

				persons * Language develops in formal and informal manner.
(3) To test the effectiveness of improvisation technique in language development of hearing impaired students.	1) There will be significant difference in pre test and post test scores for language development in the experimental group.	Control group= 19 Experimental group=21	't' statistics for Hypothesis	* No significant difference in pre test and post test scores for language development in the experimental group.
	2) There will be no significant difference in pre test and post test scores for language development in the control group.	Control group=19 Experimental group=21a	't' statistics For Hypothesis	*no significant difference in pre test and post test scores for language development in the control group.
	3) There will be a positive gain in the language development of experimental group as compared to that in control group.	Control group =19 Experimental group = 21	't' statistics for Hypothesis	* a positive gain in the language development of experimental group as compared to that in control group

CPSIA information can be obtained
at www.ICGtesting.com
Printed in the USA
LVHW052127301222
736235LV00034B/1230